T0347408

Activities in Action: Proceedings of the National Association of Activity Professionals 1990 Conference

Activities in Action: Proceedings of the National Association of Activity Professionals 1990 Conference

Phyllis M. Foster
Editor

The Haworth Press
New York • London

Activities in Action: Proceedings of the National Association of Activity Professionals 1990 Conference has also been published as *Activities, Adaptation & Aging*, Volume 15, Number 4 1991.

The Haworth Press, Inc. 10 Alice Street, Binghamton, NY 13904-1580
EUROSPAN/Haworth, 3 Henrietta Street, London WC2E 8LU England

Library of Congress Cataloging-in-Publication Data

National Association of Activity Professionals (U.S.). Convention (8th : 1990 : Seattle, Wash.)
    Activities in action : proceedings of the National Association of Activity Professionals 1990 Conference / Phyllis M. Foster, editor.
    p. cm.
    "Has also been published as Activities, adaptation & aging, volume 15, number 4 1991" — T.p. verso.
    Includes bibliographical references.
    ISBN 1-56024-132-2
    1. Occupational therapy — Congresses. 2. Nursing homes — Recreational activities — Congresses. I. Foster, Phyllis M.
II. Title.
RC953.8.O22N38 1991
618.97'58515 — dc20   990-28487
                                                                         CIP

Activities in Action: Proceedings of the National Association of Activity Professionals 1990 Conference

CONTENTS

ALL HAWORTH BOOKS & JOURNALS
ARE PRINTED ON CERTIFIED
ACID-FREE PAPER

ABOUT THE EDITOR

Phyllis M. Foster, ACC, is in private practice as the Therapeutic Activities Consultant to a number of Colorado long term care facilities. A Charter member of the National Association of Activity Professionals, she served on the original Steering Committee for formation of the autonomous association, a two-year term as Vice President, and two full terms as President. She also holds memberships in the Colorado Activity Professionals' Association and the Colorado Homes and Services for the Aged. Ms. Foster has over 25 years experience in activities as both a coordinator and a consultant. She has been involved in providing training for activity personnel in 15 states and Canada since 1970. Highly regarded in her Profession, Ms. Foster received the American Health Care Association's Better Life Award for humanitarian services in caring for the needs of the elderly in 1978 and the Colorado Health Care Association Vesta Bowden Award in 1982 for contributions to long term care through education. In 1990, the National Association of Activity Professionals presented her with their Distinguished Service Award for her contributions to the activity profession.

Preface

The National Association of Activity Professionals is the only national organization representing activity professionals in geriatric settings exclusively. It was founded by activity professionals for activity professionals and serves as a catalyst for professional and personal growth and provides a national voice on aging and long-term-care issues.

It is a pleasure to provide this special collection focusing on the NAAP 1990 Conference. We were unable to obtain all presented sessions but felt the selected articles contained within these pages, convey the overall message of both the Conference and the NAAP.

Also included at the close of this special collection is Volume 4, #1 of "The Aging and Leisure Bibliography." This is a regular feature of the publication *ACTIVITIES, ADAPTATION & AGING*, and is edited by Dr. Ted Tedrick of Temple University. While the Bibliography has no connection with the NAAP Conference, it was felt that the increased specialized readership of this particular issue would benefit from knowing the availability of this excellent resource.

Phyllis M. Foster, ACC
Editor

BOARD OF TRUSTEES
1990-1991

Reprinted by permission of The National Association of Activity Professionals, 1225 Eye Street, N.W. – Suite 300, Washington, DC 20005, (202) 289-0722 Ext. 248, Charles Price, Executive Director.

The NAAP Mission and Philosophy

The NAAP's mission is to promote standards of excellence, provide support systems, foster research, and assure educational opportunities to its members. In order to fulfill this mission the following objectives are pursued:

The improvement and promotion of activity programming.

The promotion and offering of appropriate educational opportunities, specifically geared to the activity profession, to address the needs of the people it serves.

The identification of the scope and realm of the activity profession and the activity professional.

The development of a body of knowledge, specific to activities, through research, publishing and resource review.

Promotion of the delivery of activity services through working with allied professional groups, consumer organizations, regulatory agencies and provider representatives.

Providing a support system that will assist the activity professional in career development.

Reprinted by permission of The National Association of Activity Professionals, 1225 Eye Street, N.W. — Suite 300, Washington, DC 20005, (202) 289-0722 Ext. 248, Charles Price, Executive Director.

Chronology of the NAAP

The National Association of Activity Professionals (NAAP) began with an exploratory meeting in Chicago, IL on March 21, 1981 involving 20 activity professionals from 11 states, after associations were surveyed the previous November to determine interest. At the second organizational meeting the following June 26-27, a Steering Committee accepted draft bylaws and charter memberships were opened.

On October 2-3, 1981 the NAAP held its third organizational meeting with 16 states now represented on the Steering Committee. The following December saw publication of the NAAP's first bi-monthly newsletter, then called UPDATE. By February, 1982 the NAAP began its first political action campaign against threatened federal deregulation of activities and long-term care. That same month, the national membership elected a Board of Trustees from a slate chosen at the third organizational meeting. In March, by-laws and policies were ratified by a charter membership of 254.

The first meeting of the NAAP Board of Trustees was held July 9-10, 1982 in Des Plaines, IL and the first annual NAAP convention was held April 29-30, 1983 in Cincinnati, OH. The following March, the State Contact program began and on September 23, 1983 the NAAP was chartered as a nonprofit corporation in Illinois. Two months later, the NAAP began liaison with the American Health Care Association, the first of its outreach initiatives to other interest groups.

On January 27, 1984 the first National Activity Professionals Day was celebrated. The second annual convention was in Denver, CO

Reprinted by permission of The National Association of Activity Professionals, 1225 Eye Street, N.W. – Suite 300, Washington, DC 20005, (202) 289-0722 Ext. 248, Charles Price, Executive Director.

April 26-28. On July 17, 1984 the National Activity Education organization was chartered. Formal liaison with the National Therapeutic Recreation Society (NTRS) was established in October. On December 12 the NAAP submitted a position paper on nursing home regulations to the Institute of Medicine.

In the year 1985 on April 25-27 the NAAP held its third annual convention in Buffalo, NY. In 1986 the convention was held in Sacramento, CA on April 24-26. At that convention the first NAAP awards for Distinguished Merit, Service, Excellence and Volunteer of the Year were awarded.

Between September and November 1986 the NAAP legislative committee conducted a survey on new long-term care survey procedures for input to the Health Care Financing Administration (HCFA). The NAAP Board held its first mid-year meeting October 9-10, 1986 and on October 30 the National Certification Council for Activity Professionals (NCCAP) was incorporated.

The 1987 convention was held in Chicago, IL on April 23-24. That year, thanks in part to legislative efforts by the NAAP, Congress passed legislation requiring all nursing homes that receive federal funds to have an ongoing activities program directed by a qualified professional.

In 1988 the Sixth Annual NAAP Convention was held on April 28-30 in Minneapolis, MN and the Board of Trustees decided to establish a NAAP national office in Washington, DC. Effective June 1, the management firm of Linton, Mields, Reisler and Cottone was retained to manage NAAP affairs. In September a membership drive was begun which increased membership from about 1300 to 2100 by April, 1989. The NAAP Newsletter became a monthly.

On February 2, 1989 HCFA issued new federal regulations on long-term care facilities and the NAAP began lobbying to improve the regulations and the interpretive guidelines implementing them. As a result NCCAP was acknowledged by HCFA as a recognized accrediting body for activity professionals and there were other improvements in the guidelines. Convention that year was held in Charlotte, NC April 26-29.

In November-December, 1989 the NAAP was invited by HCFA to participate in national surveyor training. During 1990 cooperative legislative efforts have been launched in concert with NTRS and the American Therapeutic Recreation Association. The NAAP is also working with other interest groups and the film industry to resolve copyright infringement liability for a nursing homes and retirement communities showing video movies.

The 1990 convention is in Seattle, WA on April 21-23.

The Eighth Annual Convention of the National Association of Activity Professionals: A Summary

Charles F. Price

Four hundred activity professionals from throughout the United States, Canada, and even as far away as Bermuda gathered in Seattle, WA during the third week of April 1990 to attend the eighth annual convention of the National Association of Activity Professionals.

They came for a variety of reasons. First and foremost, there were valuable sessions on activity programming and professional development to attend, as a way of sharpening professional skills and earning continuing education credits needed to maintain professional standing.

There were other activity practitioners with whom to share experiences, ideas, concerns, and information about professional opportunities; and this kind of peer interaction enabled conventioneers to participate in an important national support network.

There were new government requirements for long-term care to learn about, in order to comply with federal and state law governing activity practice. There were opportunities to view the exhibited products of vendors serving the activities field. And finally, there was the beautiful waterfront "Emerald City" of Seattle to enjoy.

The convention was held April 21-23 at the Seattle Sheraton Hotel and Towers. Its theme, "Sailing into the Future," symbolized both the nautical spirit of the convention site on Puget Sound and

Charles F. Price is NAAP Executive Director.

　　1

the challenges that will have to be confronted as the activity profession charts its course into the 1990's and the beyond.

Convention sessions were explicitly designed to address the issues most likely to concern the field in the immediate and long-term future. The next several years will offer much, and demand much, as the importance of activities in elderly health care is confirmed in federal and state regulation; the profession's credentialing process matures; and activity professionals further define standards of practice, ethical codes, educational requirements, and a distinct professional character.

Activity professionals won a big victory in 1987 when Congress passed a major nursing home reform law that for the first time acknowledged the importance of activities as an essential element of quality care for the elderly. That law mandated not only that there be an activity program but that there be a qualified professional directing it.

Now that the law has been enacted, it must be put into effect. The Health Care Financing Administration is in the process of writing the regulations and guidelines it will use to implement and enforce the law. Activity professionals need to be intimately familiar with these requirements, and at the NAAP convention one such regulatory instrument was given special emphasis in repeat sessions. This was the resident assessment Minimum Data Set, prepared for HCFA by private contractors as a tool for determining the condition and capabilities of residents and developing care plans.

Other session topics included reminiscence therapy, an examination of evidence showing a positive effect by activities on quality of life, relocation trauma, creative programming, adventure-based education, supervision techniques, hortitherapy, the spirituality of aging, interactive programming, one-on-one activities, overnight and day camping with long-term care residents, motivational techniques, motivation vs. burnout, programming for Alzheimers victims, educational programming, bookkeeping for consultants, and day-tripping for the elderly.

Special sessions were also held for activity professionals working in retirement living, adult day care, education, and consulting. There were also working meetings of all NAAP committees as well as the NAAP Board of Trustees.

The convention opened with a keynote address by outgoing, two-term NAAP President Phyllis M. Foster of Littleton, CO who is also editor of *Activities, Adaptation & Aging*. Ms. Foster spoke on the subject "Sailing into the '90's," discussing the future of the health care industry and the impact on the field of the federal nursing home reform amendments contained in the Omnibus Budget Reconciliation Act of 1987 (OBRA).

Closing keynoter for the convention was Denise Klein, director of the Seattle-King County Division on Aging, who spoke on the role of the professional in helping the elderly accept dependence and frailty as a natural consequence of long life.

A major convention event was the annual awards dinner and theme night, held on the evening of April 21. Conventioneers and their guests or spouses loaded on to a cruise boat to steam across Puget Sound to enjoy a salmon dinner at Kiana Lodge, a rustic ten-acre retreat located near Seattle.

During the dinner the 1990 NAAP awards were presented. Receiving the Activity Professional Award for Excellence was Ann C. Roberts, ACC of Community Convalescent Center in Riverside, CA. The Distinguished Service Award was presented to outgoing president Phyllis Foster.

Fr. Declan Madden of St. Frances Heights, Denver, CO received the Distinguished Merit Award and Alan F. Dill of Orangegrove Rehabilitation Hospital, Garden Grove, CA was given the Administrator of the Year Award. The Activity Volunteer of the Year Award went to a group of law enforcement officers from Shasta County, CA who carry out a musical ministry at Shasta Convalescent Hospital, Redding, CA. They are called the Singin' Sheriffs.

Convention participants and spouses also took advantage of other outside activities during convention week. Tours were available of downtown Seattle, Pioneer Square, the International District, and Pike Place Market; Seattle's underground; the Boeing plant; and Snoqualmie Falls/Chateau Ste. Michelle Winery.

State activity associations from around the country generously helped sponsor the convention, and their support was acknowledged during the proceedings. State sponsors included the Colorado Activity Professionals' Association; the Maryland Activity Coordinators' Society, Inc.; the Michigan Association of Activity Professionals; the Southern California Council of Activity Coordinators; and the Resident Activity Personnel in Ohio.

Support was also provided by the Connecticut Association of Therapeutic Recreation Directors; the Pennsylvania Activity Professional; the Arizona Association of Activity Professionals Association; the Florida Health Care Activity Coordinator Association; and the North Dakota Council of Activity Coordinators. Continuing education credits were available for attendance at educational sessions during the convention. The National Certification Council for Activity Professionals recognized 15 1/2 credits for attendance, while the National Continuing Education Review Service of the National Association of Boards of Examiners for Nursing Home Administrators approved the convention program for 15 clock hours of continuing education credit.

Following the closing keynote address on April 23, the final day of convention, the NAAP Annual Meeting was held, during which new officers and trustees were formally installed.

NAAP Keynote Address

Phyllis M. Foster

Welcome, Activity Professionals, to Seattle. Welcome to the 8th annual conference of the National Association of Activity Professionals. Our local arrangements committee's months of hard work have paid off, and we are here to celebrate Sailing into the Future.

This lovely city so close to the sea is the perfect place to meet and discuss the smooth as well as the rough waters we have traveled and still have to travel.

We are about to install Jane Carlson as our new president and to welcome several newly elected trustees who bring new talents and new expertise to the Board of Trustees. Ideas they already have are exciting. I want to thank all of the board members who have served during my two terms as President. You richly deserve all of our thanks and praise.

For you have helped guide the National Association of Activity Professionals (the NAAP) through the most critical times of its young life. Those of you who previously served on the board of trustees will recall that we have thought each year was the hardest one we had ever faced and the next could only be easier.

But so far, the challenges keep getting tougher and they keep on coming. There is no coasting when you are building an association

Phyllis M. Foster, ACC, is a Therapeutic Activities Consultant in private practice in Colorado and is Editor of the professional journal, *Activities, Adaption & Aging*. A Charter Member of the National Association of Activity Professionals, she served on the original Steering Committee for formation of the association, a two year term as Vice President (1984-1986) and two full terms as President (1986-1990). Phyllis has been involved in activities with geriatric clients for more than 25 years. Correspondence should be addressed to Phyllis M. Foster, 6549 S. Lincoln Street, Littleton, CO 80121-2325.

This speech was prepared for delivery at Seattle, WA, April 21, 1990.

like the NAAP. There are more opportunities every day and every year, and so far we have had the energetic members and the leaders to keep going after evermore exciting goals. I say more power to us. Being cautious is not going to get us the professional recognition and status we want and need. Hard work and risktaking can and will.

The first risk that this association took was just in getting it started, and that was a big risk. In 1983 at the first NAAP conference that was held in Cincinnati, the gauntlet was thrown down in the form of a challenge by our keynote speaker.

Janice Caldwell was at that time Commissioner for Services to the Aged and Disabled at the Texas Department of Human Resources. The title of her address was "Model Homes and Master Keys." Her message to us was that activities is one of the master keys to model homes and that people were beginning to realize that activity leaders and activity programs make the crucial difference in aging with quality.

She went on to say that doing nice things for people was no longer enough. We needed to increase our educational requirements. We needed to develop standards for performance, and we needed to initiate seven-day programming—before someone else did it for us.

Janice Caldwell challenged us as an association to make the case that activities were no longer a soft expendable item, but rather that activity services were not only cost effective but cost beneficial. She further stated that the establishment of a national organization was a major first step and that we should proceed to sell ourselves and our services by being involved in and staying on top of legislative and political issues.

I believe the membership and the board of trustees accepted Janice Caldwell's challenge. The board has directed its attention since then to having a political presence on issues related to our work or to the recipients of our services. Under the very capable leadership of our Vice President/Government Relations Chair, NAAP has, in the past four years, propelled itself into the legislative arena. We owe much to Ruth Perschbacher for putting us into that arena, and I would ask you NOW to join me in acknowledging her contributions to our organization and our profession.

The written reports in your program book offer a detailed look at accomplishments that were realized through the efforts of the Government Relations Committee. But it makes me proud, and I hope it makes you proud, to know that an activity program provided by a qualified activity professional is not just a requirement. It's in federal law.

That HCFA, the Health Care Financing Administration, acknowledges the NCCAP certification process in its interpretive guidelines. That the National Therapeutic Recreation Society acknowledged the NCCAP certification process in a policy statement.

As a result of our talks together, doors have been opened between the NAAP, the NTRS and ATRA, the American Therapeutic Recreation Association, for presenting a consolidated joint recommendation for changes in the activities section of the federal final rule on Long Term Care.

I remind you that there is strength in numbers. We've said that from the very beginning of this association and it can't be emphasized enough. The larger we grow, the more vocal we can become. The more we can achieve. (The full text of the Long Term Care recommendation is in the appendix of this article, page 14.)

I'm proud to know that the NAAP has held a leadership position in the discussion related to the showing of VCR movies in nursing homes and any other facilities which provide long-term care. (A full report on the 10-year agreement, with a section of questions and answers, is in the appendix of this article, page 18.)

It makes me proud that we received an invitation from HCFA to participate in and conduct surveyor training on activities programming. Two of our board members, Ruth Perschbacher as Government Relations Chair and Jane Carlson as Standards Chair and now President Elect, conducted the activities section of the surveyor training, and they received very positive feedback from both HCFA and the individual surveyors. When the federally mandated resident assessment appears at your facility, you can take pride in knowing that the activities section was not written solely by someone from another discipline as has happened so frequently in the past. Your national association has had a strong role in the final writing of that assessment.

I'm not going to belabor our many successes. As I said earlier, detail is in your program book. But what I do hope you realize is that there is a direct correlation between our accomplishments and our move to the nation's capitol. While those accomplishments were initiated and guided by our Government Relations Committee, the lobbying, support and on-site availability of our professional staff saw our contributions truly impact the system.

That move to Washington was yet another risk, another challenge, and it was undertaken during my watch. Circumstances had put us in a position of having to move our central office out of a private home. And it was at the 1988 convention in Minnesota that the Board of Trustees voted unanimously to move the NAAP headquarters to Washington, D.C., under an association management contract with Linton, Mields, Reisler & Cottone, Ltd. Yes, a costly venture. But a very wise venture.

We draw on LMRC's expertise and time under a contract which gives us a certain number of hours from each area. There is staff support for our volunteer labors in a number of subject areas, and we are taking full advantage of it—and more.

We have already undertaken many new ideas and projects and expanded so many existing ones that we are stretching our capacity. Taking stock of the time spent has shown how far we have come—and how far we must now go to build on our success. As anticipated, that move has served to increase the visibility and recognition of activity professionals by providing direct contact with appropriate organizations and individuals. As a result, the NAAP is now being represented on Washington-based committees and referred to as a group to be acknowledged, included and considered.

We owe much to our executive director Charles Price for helping us get to that point in our life. For some of us who have enjoyed donating our time to hands-on work for our profession through the NAAP, the transition to more and more work being turned over to the management team in Washington is a tough one. Even though that is an expensive route, that we will all have to help in financing, it is necessary to ensure our future.

We are leaders in a growing industry in an increasingly complex professional scene. As individuals we are getting busier and busier and are beginning to outrun our own personal resources.

This national organization is less than 10 years old, but it has a phenomenal record of success in federal legislative issues, in membership growth, and in building recognition for our profession. I am not just talking to you here today about this transition in our organization.

It has been on the agenda of the board meetings this week, and it has been on the minds of all of the officers for months. It is a serious turning point for the NAAP. The key to success now is in expanding our base and our numbers and our financial capacity. When you really think about it, for $45 you are getting a lot.

Current financial circumstances have triggered numerous Ways and Means initiatives that have helped provide us the resources necessary to continue. You as members have a responsibility to let us hear from you. We need to know what you're thinking and where you want us to go. Can we increase our commitment, knowing that increases in costs go with it? Do we believe enough in the NAAP?

There is one more initiative by activity professionals which I believe would lead to quantum improvement in the status of our profession. That is to have a closer working relationship between state and local associations and the national association. It is not just the shared interests. It is not just the combined clout in terms of numbers. It is a whole which could be greater than the sum of the parts.

In my home state of Colorado the combined clout of the state and national associations helped us impact state regulatory changes. I am convinced that the prestige of the national association backing our state efforts made the decisive difference. National and state organizations working together could make us a formidable group, and I believe it is only a matter of time until we achieve a solid working relationship. Won't you help me with the groundwork here and now?

Our Ways and Means Chairman Brad Beckman initiated state sponsorships this year to help get us over a hump, and the response was very good. Fourteen states responded to that initiative and between them they donated nearly $5000.

These states recognized that while our membership is on an individual basis, the actions taken by this national association benefit all activity professionals, whether they are members or not. Those states recognize the value of our national presence.

I challenge all of you to introduce the state sponsorship program in your state. This program could be a good first step toward state and national association cooperation. It could lead to a meaningful formal relationship between the groups. The networking is needed just as much as the revenue.

That in a nutshell tells you where we are now, and it's apparent that if we want to continue to have a say in how our profession is regulated there is no turning back now. Our future will be written for us if we slip back into the past. But this time we are in a position to chart our own direction.

The challenge that this association will face in the 1990s includes staying involved with the other Washington based associations who are establishing training for the OBRA requirements. We must also continue our participation in surveyor training and work towards activity professionals being represented on surveyor teams.

We must develop a college curriculum for activities, starting with a two-year community college associate degree. We must pursue the ultimate goal of establishing degree programs at a full four-year college level and perhaps someday even building that discipline to include post-graduate academic programs. It is possible and we have the clout to do it.

We must strengthen and improve opportunities for continuing education courses for those practicing activity professionals who want to update their skills. There is much work in this area for the NAAP to undertake: devising a means of accrediting continuing education courses, developing course materials, and maintaining an information clearinghouse on available programs.

Public education offers more challenges for our profession. What we do and who we are has been a well-kept secret, and it is to our advantage now to change that. One thing I would like to share is a personal goal of mine—to have a local activity association representative at every "career night" held by a school district and at every job fair held by a city or state. It is something you can do within your state or local association. It can be done.

Staff ratios is another area where the NAAP must increase its efforts if HCFA disallows that portion of the joint recommendation we submitted with NTRS and ATRA. A national activities association is the proper place for conducting research and the studies necessary for determining an equitable ratio of activity staff to residents. The NAAP can then assist state associations in selling that ratio to their state regulatory agencies.

Government's role in health care is going to be defined by the number crunchers during the 90s unless organizations like the NAAP stay in there and argue for the human side — the quality of care side and the cost effectiveness of keeping older Americans not just comfortable but engaged in life. We have a large task, as leaders of our profession, in shaping a strong message. No one can do that for us. However, the role of professional lobbying staff in delivering our message is growing by leaps and bounds.

Adult day care, retirement living, long term care facilities — all geriatric settings where activity professionals work — are spread out geographically, just as our association is. It is a ready-made marketing network that few organizations have at their disposal.

The NAAP's tracking of national legislation is outstanding, and the NAAP's record of generating comment from members on issues of interest is remarkably good. NAAP members have a commitment to building our profession.

When we look at the response we get from a call to our members, we are reminded of that commitment. In a mailing to a general audience, a group should be pleased with a response of 4 to 6 percent. In a mailing to its own members, 10 to 12 percent is considered normal.

Our response percentage in the mailing of our bylaws — and let's face it, reading bylaws takes a lot of doing — was 20 percent of the membership. For some of us that sounds like a small number, but when you look at the norm, it is a remarkable performance.

NAAP, during its first 8 years of life, went from a beginning task force to true organization to major national coalition member in almost giant steps. It did so by sheer will of its board members and organizing committee. NAAP came together because activity professionals in a number of states recognized the need for combined clout — and pooled their efforts at the right time. If they had tried too soon, they might have failed. Or waiting too late, their efforts might have been too little.

Timing and talent made us launch a winner. And the progress since then has gone on by sheer determination. There are no national organizations who are players in congressional issues with dues of $45 per year, with large membership in only a few states, and with total membership at less than 2200. But NAAP did and NAAP is. NAAP goes into the 1990s playing catch up with its own agenda. Advice we are receiving in and out of the organization tells us to stick with our commitment to a Washington presence and make the sacrifices needed to maintain that strong presence.

Being an organization started in our own time, we have a unity of purpose which has by itself helped us through many storms. We are emerging stronger and more confident. We deserve to take our places with other groups of professional care givers.

The assistance and support of the full-time staff has allowed the Board of Trustees to realize a number of goals. The most obvious has been the expansion of NAAP News to monthly publication, strengthening our direct communication link with our members.

In the next few years, this will become a very significant professional organization. Being an early leader of NAAP will one day be a high honor to recall. Though it seems now that it is all uphill work to gain recognition as a professional and as a skilled worker deserving of better wages and benefits, we will look back in a few years and see battles won. Stature gained. More coalitions coming to us for advice and help. Membership numbers more in line with the number of practicing activity professionals.

We are one of the great bargains of 1990 — for 87 cents a week you get a Washington office, lobbying on behalf of your professional issues, plus representation at the meetings of national coalition working groups, a monthly newsletter, and hundreds of hours of top-notch work from the staff and the all-volunteer board of the NAAP.

If it sounds like a commercial, it is one. Our progress so far has come from a combination of very hard work, very timely actions, and very good luck. To sustain that progress and help our profession come of age, we must now build our numbers — members and membership numbers make the long-term difference.

It takes a national organization to marshall the resources needed to carry on this type of fight on behalf of individual practitioners. Many groups like activity professionals are finding it necessary to join the battles. It is hard work, expensive work, but it is paying off.

I believe philosophical questions are going to dominate the agenda in conferences of activity professionals like this one over the next year or two. Questions of philosophical direction surface in every discussion we have about how to improve our professional image.

Philosophical winds of change are always blowing through professions which are growing. If we want to avoid change, we will have to settle for its tradeoff which is stagnation. And I do not detect among activity professionals great support for the status quo.

On the one hand, there is a move to define and measure more precisely the work of activity professionals. This can be a plus. In addition, when we measure our work we are more likely to be called "activity therapists" in the staff directory. For many of our practitioners that would be an immediate increase in prestige.

Our practitioners want professional development opportunities as individuals and as a group. But at the same time we want that professional progress to take place on a human scale. We want to quantify our results with residents of long-term care facilities—but we want to do so in a way that allows taking into account the resident community as a whole as well as the individual patient needs. That is the traditional approach of activity professionals, and I freely admit that I am a traditionalist.

I came into this association as an activity director. I am committed to the notion that I can do more for the residents of a facility by developing an environment that encourages continued participation in living than I can as a deliverer of individual therapy schemes of certain duration—undertaken by prescription.

Quality of life elements should not be subject to limitation. They should be ongoing. Food does not cease after a certain number of meals have been served. Food for the mind and soul should not either. It is easier to sell federal regulators on the "measured therapy" approach to activities, but how do you keep the quality of life measures sensitive enough to read one person's self-esteem.

Our anxiety to show that our care elements are more than amusements and diversions for older people are leading us into this trap of rigid clinical decisions. There is a great lure to the arguments on both sides of this discussion. And both sides believe that their path will lead to more professional recognition and better pay status.

This is a dilemma we are only beginning to face; it will be important to us for some time to come.

But in one way or another, almost all of the concerns I have listed are only differing aspects of the same overriding goal. The goal is to see universal acceptance of the activity profession as a legitimate, vital, and respected member of the elderly health-care team. By that I mean that our calling should command from other care-giving professionals, from providers and federal regulators and state surveyors, and from residents and their families and the public at large, an acknowledgement that what we do has an affect on psycho-social and physical well being that can be demonstrated and that is crucial to the life quality of the elderly in our care.

That kind of acknowledgement will lead to higher salaries, improved working conditions, opportunities for advancement, and all the other benefits a true professional status confers. The progress we have made to this point gives us reason to hope that in the 1990s we can achieve this goal.

Appendix I

NAAP/NTRS/ATRA Recommendations on Long-Term Care Sent to HCFA

As was reported in the March issue of NAAP News, the NAAP has been working with the National Therapeutic Recreation Society and the American Therapeutic Recreation Association in recent weeks to develop a joint set of recommendations to the Health Care Financing Administration on needed revisions in the federal regulations governing long-term care facilities and the interpretive guidelines used by surveyors to evaluate the adequacy of care in such facilities.

Early in March the recommendations were finalized and forwarded to HCFA. The text appears on this page. The proposals were developed in consultation with Government Relations Chair Ruth Perschbacher and the NAAP Executive Council. In addition to those whose names appear in the statement, others contributing materially to this cooperative effort included Dr. Fred Humphrey, immediate past president of NTRS and Yvonne Washington, former NTRS executive director.

Consolidated Recommendations for Changes in the Activities Section of the Final Rule of the Long Term Care Regulation

Submitted by
The American Therapeutic Recreation Association
The National Association of Activity Professionals
The National Therapeutic Recreation Society

The following are recommended changes for the "Activities" section, (f) under 483.15 Quality of Life, of the Final Rule for Long Term Care, as requested by the above named organizations. These changes ensure a high standard for the provision of quality services for residents.

1. a. We recommend that item 283.15 (f) (2) (iv), "has completed a training course approved by the state," *be deleted* from the regulation. This requirement is of extreme concern to us and was part of all prior correspondence and comments upon the proposed regulations, by all three organizations. Its vagueness is likely to result in inadequate amounts of training for activities personnel, placing the quality of activity programming and resident services in jeopardy.

    b. That item 283.15 (f) (2) (ii), "has 2 years experience in a social or recreational program within the last 5 years, 1 of which was full-time in a patient activities program in a health care setting," *be deleted* from the regulation. This requirement has resulted in inadequate training for activities personnel, as our organizations find so prevalent at this time. We receive phone calls from individuals daily, who have only experience to rely on, and when put in the position of "Director of Activities" require outside consultation to be able to fulfill duties such as assessment, documentation and quality assurance, to name a few. This criterion is acceptable for additional Activities staff, however is insufficient for the Director's position.

    c. That there be an *addition* to section 283.15 (f) (2) of the regulation, stating the following:

      ii. _____ Is a qualified activity professional who is eligible for certification as an activity professional by a recognized accrediting body on August 1, 1989, or. . . .

This addition distinguishes between a therapeutic recreation specialist and an activities professional. Both are distinct professions, with separate credentialing bodies and separate competency requirements. Both of these professionals, however, work with the Activities departments of nursing homes.

2. The *addition* of a mandate requiring a Resident's Council within every nursing home. Although Family/Resident Councils are addressed with the quality of Life Standard of the regulations, the content is weak and will attain limited results. In addition, a separate mandate should be included, requiring the Administration to respond to Council concerns within two weeks of their receipt. Only with this kind of regulation can we begin to ensure empowerment for the residents in nursing homes.

3. The *addition* of a third requirement to section 483.15 (f):

(3) An Activities staff/resident ratio of 1/50.

At this time, there are facilities with Activities staff to resident ratios of 1/120 or higher. This is an extremely unrealistic task for any individual to carry out, particularly in light of the documentation requirements that accompany this position. Although the ration of 1/50 still remains high, it ensures that the Activities staff can at least impact the quality of life of nursing home residents. Ratios any higher cannot possibly be cost effective because they cannot produce the desired results.

In addition to the above requested changes in the Final Rule of Regulation, the following additional recommendations pertaining to the Interpretive Guidelines are being made. In this way, it can be ensured that continuity exists between the guideline and the regulation.

1. The following changes are recommended under *Interpretive Guideline 483.15 (f) (1)*;

a. That the statement "An activities program could address and contain the following therapeutic activities" *be restated* as the following:

"An activities program *should result in* the following therapeutic *outcomes.*" It should address and contain a wide variety of activities, as determined by the needs and interests of the resident.

b. That the following statements should *replace* the current **maintenance, empowerment, and supportive** clauses of section 483.17 (f) (1) of the guidelines:

Supportive outcomes, as evidenced by resident participation in activities which provide stimulation or solace.

Maintenance outcomes, as evidenced by resident participation in activities that promote physical, cognitive, social and/or emotional health.

Restorative outcomes, as evidenced by resident participation activities that focus on enhancing the physical and psychosocial status of the resident.

Empowerment outcomes which promote self-respect, as evidenced by resident participation in activities providing opportunities for self-expression, personal responsibility, and choice.

Evidence of these outcomes should be noted within the progress note of each resident.

2. The following changes are recommended in regards to qualified activities staff:

a. That the statement "a recognized accrediting body includes but is not limited to certification by the National Certification Council for Activity Professionals" *be deleted* from section 483.15 (f) (1).

b. That the following statement *be added* under section 483.15 (f) (2): "A recognized accrediting body includes but is not limited to the National Council for Therapeutic Recreation Certification and the National Certification Council for Activity Professionals."

3. We recommend the following *additions* under *Survey Procedures and Probes, 483.15 (f) (1)*:

a. The *addition* of a clarifier within the subsection for sampled residents who are unable to respond to questions. This should be added to the following probe:

   — Do all residents receive activities (including individual/bedside activity if warranted)?

b. The *addition* of the following two survey procedures:

   — Random observations of activity programs shall take place, including both group activity and individual or bedside activity.

   — An interview shall be conducted with the Activities staff, to complement observations and chart reviews.

We thank you for your time and consideration. Should you have further questions, please contact one of the individuals listed below:

Karen Vecchione (202) 563-8100
American Therapeutic Recreation Association

Charles Price (202) 289-0722 ext. 248

Ruth Perschbacher (704) 298-7357
National Association of Activity Professionals

Christie Cullinan (703) 820-4940
National Therapeutic Recreation Society

Appendix II

Video Movie Dispute Settled

Nursing Homes Granted 10-Year Viewing Rights

Charles F. Price

NAAP Executive Director

Months of negotiations involving NAAP, nursing home interests, répresentatives of the motion picture industry, and Congressional members and staff paid off August 3 when a settlement was announced in the years-long dispute over whether nursing homes must purchase licenses to show video movies to residents.

The agreement grants 10-year license-free viewing rights to "nursing homes, hospices, hospitals, retirement homes or other such group homes that provide long-term health or health-related care and services to individuals on a regular basis and serve as a home or residence for such individuals."

The non-legislative solution was crafted by Rep. Robert W. Kastenmeier (D-WI), Chairman of the House Judiciary Subcommittee on Courts, Intellectual Property and the Administration of Justice, which has jurisdiction over matters relating to video movie copyrights. Kastenmeier had held a subcommittee hearing on the controversy April 5, and afterward set out to reconcile the opposing views of the parties.

His agreement incorporates concepts previously hammered out by NAAP, the American Association of Homes for the Aging, the American Health Care Association, the Motion Picture Association of America, and three licensing organizations in a long series of meetings last winter and spring held under the auspices of Sen. William Roth (R-DE) and Rep. Benjamin Cardin (D-MD), who had each offered legislation intended to solve the video movie licensing problem. The Kastenmeier solution also includes elements of the Roth and Cardin bills.

Facilities covered by the agreement, under the term "nursing homes" as defined above, would not include every wing of a hospital in which only one section may be a nursing home dedicated to long-term health care for the elderly and the remaining wings are dedicated to short-term or even out-patient treatment for the community at large.

If the "nursing home" is located on the grounds of a hospital, retirement or residential community or other facility, the rights conferred by the agreement would only cover performances in the nursing home itself in a common area serving the nursing home residents. Not covered are large condominiums or retirement complexes where residents live independently in private units and do not regularly receive health-related services. The settlement was announced at a Capitol Hill press conference called by Rep. Kastenmeier, who acknowledged in his statement the participation of NAAP and the other parties in helping reach a satisfactory agreement. Sen Roth also publicly thanked NAAP and the other groups for their contributions to the settlement.

Accepting the agreement on behalf of the movie industry were Warner Brothers, Paramount, Columbia, Buena Vista (Disney), MCA, Orion, MGM/UA, 20th Century Fox, and Turner. Also accepting were the three major licensing firms, Motion Picture Licensing Corporation (MPLC), Swank, and Films, Inc.

It was the aggressive marketing tactics of MPLC that first raised concerns in the nursing home community about the fairness of requiring public-performances licenses for showing video movies in long-term care facilities, which are in all respects the homes of the residents.

The agreement becomes binding by the writing of $10 checks from AAHA and AHCA to charities designated by the movie studios, including Ronald McDonald House, Better World Society, American Foundation for AIDS research, American Cancer Society, National Multiple Sclerosis Society, and the Will Rogers Institute.

The agreement expires December 31, 2001 and covers performances that may have previously taken place in nursing homes. The period is thought to be long enough to permit stability but sufficiently short to reevaluate the technology as it develops further. The Congressional sponsors originally favored a five-year term, which is the typical sunset period for copyright legislation.

The Video Movie Agreement
Questions and Answers

Which long-term care facilities are covered?

1. Nursing Homes. Traditional nursing home settings are covered regardless of whether the residents are elderly. Residential mental health centers and intermediate care facilities for the mentally retarded (ICF/MRs) also are included.

2. Personal Care Homes and Homes for the Aging. These facilities are completely covered by the agreement.

3. Continuing Care Retirement Communities. The nursing home components of CCRCs are completely covered, even if the film is shown in a

common area of the independent living unit or wing, as long as that common area is serving nursing home residents. Independent living wings of CCRCs are covered if the residents on that wing also receive long-term health or health-related care and services. Examples of health related services which were discussed during negotiation of the agreements include combinations of health monitoring and screening, physical examinations, on-call medical or nursing personnel, personal care services, nutrition consultation and special meals, transportation to medical appointments, home care visits, and the like. The Congressional sponsors of the agreement have clearly stated that the agreement does not apply to large condominium or retirement complexes where residents live independently in private units and do not regularly receive health-related services.

Personal care units in CCRCs are completely covered.

4. What kind of technology can be used to show films? The agreement provides that films may be shown with videocassette records on television sets like those commonly used in a private home. This is in line with the intent of the Congressional sponsors that nursing home residents retain the rights they enjoyed in their own homes. Wide screen TVs and other advanced technology will be protected under the agreement to the extent that they are used by ordinary household consumers in your community.

5. What about showing films through closed-circuit television? The agreements do not protect the use of closed-circuit television or any other "re-transmission" methods.

6. Can fees be charged to residents or others to view the film? The facility may not make a direct charge for or otherwise derive commercial advantage from showing the films.

7. What should facilities say if they are contacted in the future by a motion picture licensing organization and asked to license their beds or units? Facilities meeting the definition of a nursing home in the agreement should tell the licensing organization that their activities involving films conform to the August 3, 1990 agreement with the studios.

If a facility or wing of a facility which is not covered by the agreement shows videos and is contacted by a licensing organization, it is likely that the facility would be asked to "cease and desist" its video activity or become licensed. If the facility chooses to continue showing the films without a license, the studio or distributor may choose to sue.

(Adapted with permission from material prepared by the American Association of Homes for the Aging)

Federally Mandated
Nursing Home Resident Assessment:
Implications
for Activity Professionals

Ruth Perschbacher

SUMMARY. Quality of life for individual nursing home residents has become a primary focus for nursing home care. Providing this quality begins with a comprehensive assessment which identifies resident strengths and preferences. The federally mandated resident assessment provides a format for interdisciplinary assessments and care plans which are individualized and resident centered. Activity professionals will play a key role in this assessment and its emphasis on the quality of life aspects of residents' lives.

Ruth Perschbacher, ACC, RMT-BC, served as Vice President and Government Relations Chair for the National Association of Activity Professionals (NAAP) from 1986-1990. She served as a representative of the NAAP on the Federal Resident Assessment Advisory Committee. She is the owner of Bristlecone Consulting Company and can be reached at Route 2, Box 458, Asheville, NC 28805.

Parts of this paper have been published in the Tennessee Health Care Association's quarterly magazine, *Perspective*, Winter 1990 Issue.

References in this article which pertain to the Minimum Data Set, the Activities Care Plan Module, and the Resident Assessment Protocols are based on the most recent materials available to the author. Final formats and specifications regarding publishing of these materials had not been established at deadline. These materials were developed under contract with the Health Care Financing Administration, contract no. 500-88-0055. Address correspondence to John N. Morris, PhD, Department of Social Gerontological Research, Hebrew Rehabilitation Center for Aged, 1200 Centre Street, Boston, MA 02131.

OVERVIEW

On December 22, 1987, Congress passed a federal law[1] which represented the most dramatic legislative changes in nursing home regulation since the mid-70's. For the first time in federal nursing home law, "quality of life" was recognized as a key component of nursing home care. Previous regulations and laws had not specified this as a necessary requirement or expectation. Congress's commitment that quality of life becomes a reality for nursing home residents was exemplified in the law's mandate that a federal nursing home resident assessment tool be developed.

Establishment of a federal assessment tool grew out of the findings of the Institute of Medicine's (IOM) Committee on Nursing Home Regulations which published its report, *Improving the Quality of Nursing Homes* in 1986. The report established the importance of assessment to the care planning process, outcomes of care, facility management of quality care, and regulatory functions (Institute of Medicine, 1986). The IOM Committee noted that uniform assessment data on resident status and changes of status would facilitate a change in focusing the survey process and care delivery on outcomes of care rather than on specific facility procedures.

DEVELOPMENT OF THE RESIDENT ASSESSMENT

The Omnibus Budget Reconciliation Act of 1987 (OBRA '87) required the Secretary of Health and Human Services to develop this assessment process by October of 1990. Under this legislative mandate, each nursing facility certified by Medicare and Medicaid must conduct a "comprehensive, accurate, standardized, reproducible assessment of each resident's functional capacities." This assessment is to describe the "resident's capability to perform daily life functions and significant impairments in functional capacity" and is to be based on a "uniform minimum data set." On February 2, 1989, the Secretary of Health and Human Services published the minimum data set in the Federal Register. "The comprehensive

---

1.(Nursing Home Reform Section of the Omnibus Budget Reconciliation (OBRA) Act of 1987, commonly referred to as OBRA 87.)

assessment must include at least the following information: medically defined conditions and prior medical history, medical status measurement, functional status, sensory and physical impairments, nutritional status and requirements, special treatments or procedures, psychosocial status, discharge potential, dental condition, activities potential, rehabilitation potential, cognitive status, and drug therapy" (Department of Health and Human Services, 1989).

The Health Care Financing Administration (HCFA), which establishes regulations for nursing homes, contracted with the Research Triangle Institute and its subcontractors, Hebrew Rehabilitation Center for Aged, Brown University, and the University of Michigan, to develop and evaluate a resident assessment system. While it is anticipated that most states will follow the resident assessment developed by this team, individual states may develop their own assessment process as long as it is based on the minimum data set established by the Secretary as well as any other requirements HCFA may establish.

The Research Triangle team have developed a resident assessment tool which consists of three parts: the minimum data set for nursing facility resident assessment and care screening (MDS), resident assessment protocols, and care plan modules. This process links assessment and care planning into a circular process where one leads into the other. The MDS is based on the areas the Secretary specified and is designed to capture the "minimum" number of items needed to begin a comprehensive assessment. The MDS provides a care planning foundation which recognizes the resident as an individual with diverse physical, emotional, and social needs. While many aspects of the MDS focus on the functional status of the resident, other items deal with individual preferences such as customary routines and activities. The MDS provides a holistic view of individual residents and assists in identification of how a resident's strengths and needs in one area affect other areas of his/her life (Morris, J.N. et al., 1990).

Resident assessment protocols (RAPs) consist of "triggers" and related guidelines. The triggers are based on the MDS and should lead staff to more care planning and/or assessment in specific areas. The guidelines assist staff in determining where these care planning approaches should be focused. The guidelines encourage exploration of approaches which relate to the triggers, i.e., what other areas of the MDS may relate to this trigger? What further information should be obtained? For example, the MDS identifies a resident who is severely cognitively impaired. The "trigger" lists the specific item or items on the MDS which relate to severe cognitive impairment as well as related problems such as incontinence, wandering, use of restraints, etc. The RAP guidelines would provide information about how this resident could be optimally served in the least restrictive environment.

Care planning modules have also been developed to provide long term care professionals with data about the "state of the art" in care planning. These modules provide educational guidelines for staff to use in implementing the resident assessment process. They are not intended to be prescriptive, but are to provide useful information which will enhance care planning practices.

Extensive research, clinical review, and revision have been a part of the assessment's development. This tool's evolution has been a participatory process. Its holistic intent has been reflected in the involvement of a number of individuals from a variety of disciplines, including nursing, social work, geriatric and rehabilitative medicine, psychiatry, psychology, physical therapy, occupational therapy, speech therapy, activities, dietetics, and others. Consumers, advocates, providers, regulators, researchers, and experts in measurement have also taken part in this project.

RESIDENT ASSESSMENT'S RELATION TO ACTIVITIES

"Activity potential" was defined in the Department of Health and Human Services' State Operations Manual for federal surveyors (Department of Health and Human Services, 1989) as "the resident's ability and desire to take part in activity pursuits which maintain or improve physical, mental, and psychosocial well-being. Activity pursuits refer to any activity outside of ADL's which a person pursues in order to obtain a sense of well-being. [This] also includes activities which provide benefits in the areas of self-esteem, pleasure, comfort, health, education, creativity, success, and financial or emotional independence. The assessment should consider the resident's normal everyday routines and lifetime preferences." This definition provides a foundation for establishing activity assessments and care planning.

The MDS section which is most specifically related to activity assessment (Department of Health and Human Services, 1990) is entitled "Activity Pursuit Patterns" (Diagram A). This section (I) has five categories. The first category (1) focuses on the amount of time the resident is awake during the morning, afternoon, and evening. The second category (2) identifies the resident's average time involvement in activities as most, some, little or none. The third category (3) lists four preferred activity settings: own room, day/activity room, inside nursing home/off unit, and/or outside facility. The fourth category (4) has a listing of general activities' prefer-

SECTION I. ACTIVITY PURSUIT PATTERNS

1.	TIME AWAKE	(Check appropriate time periods—last 7 days) Resident awake all or most of time (i.e., no naps or naps no more than one hour per time period) in the:			
		Morning	a.	Evening	c.
		Afternoon	b.	NONE OF ABOVE	d.
2.	AVERAGE TIME INVOLVED IN ACTIVITIES	(Code correct response) 0. Most 1. Some	2. Little 3. None		
3.	PREFERRED ACTIVITY SETTINGS	(Check all settings in which activities are preferred)			
		Own room	a.	Outside facility	d
		Day/activity room	b.	NONE OF ABOVE	e
		Inside NH/off unit	c.		
4.	GENERAL ACTIVITIES PREFER-ENCES (adapted according to resident's current abilities)	(Check all specific activity preferences)			
		Cards/other games	a.	Spiritual/religious activ.	f
		Crafts/arts	b.	Trips/shopping	g
		Exercise	c.	Walking/wheeling outdoors	h
		Music	d.		
		Read/write	e.	Watch TV	i
				NONE OF ABOVE	j
5.	PREFERS MORE OR DIFFERENT ACTIVITIES	Resident expresses/indicates preference for other activities/choices. 0. No 1. Yes			

Diagram A

ences adapted according to resident's current abilities. Those prefer-ences are: cards/other games, crafts/arts, exercise, music, read/write, spiritual/religious activities, trips/shopping, walking/wheeling out-doors, and/or watching TV. The fifth category (5) indicates a resi-dent's preference for more or different activities.

The Activities Resident Assessment Protocol (Department of Health and Human Services, 1990) uses these Activity Pursuit Pat-terns' categories to "trigger" residents who need further activity care planning. For example, a resident who is awake much of the day (Category 1), but has little or no time in activity involvement (Category 2) would be "triggered" since further evaluation needs to be done to identify why this resident has low involvement. An-other example would be a resident who prefers more or different activity choices (Category 5). Further assessment would be needed to discover what types of activities this resident would prefer, and care planning would need to identify approaches which would facil-itate this resident's participation in these activities.

Many other areas of the MDS are applicable to activities "trig-gers." Some examples are residents who have poor communication and/or poor hearing, visual deficits, severely impaired cognitive skills, unsettled relationships, etc. An example of a trigger which involves the activity pursuit section and other sections would be a resident who has little or no involvement in activities (Category 2), is withdrawn, and has good short term memory (other sections of the MDS). The Activities RAP directs the activity professional to pursue whether the resident is suitably challenged or over stimu-lated, if the resident has had a recent decline in functioning, if the presence of environmental or health factors could impact on activity involvement, and/or if there have been any changes in availability of family/friends/staff support. Under each area, the Activities RAP provides further information and questions. For example, under "Is resident suitably challenged/over stimulated?", the RAP states "To some extent, competence depends on environmental demands. When the challenge is not demanding enough, the resident can become bored, perhaps withdrawn, may resort to daydreaming, fault-finding, may even behave mischievously to relieve the boredom . . ." Examples of questions are: "Do current activity levels correspond to resident values, attitudes, and lifetime expectations? Does the resident consider 'leisure activities' a waste of time? . . . " It is also important to review the MDS background information which is taken only at admission. This includes such items as birth date, lifetime occupation, marital status, etc. These certainly are relevant to activity care planning. Perhaps one of the most valuable areas to study is the "Customary Routine" section. This section provides a picture of the resident's daily life patterns before entering the long term care facility. Data about resident preferences with regard to use of time, for example, "stays busy with hobbies, reading, or fixed daily routine," and "stays up late at night" provide clues to scheduling of group or individual activities. Preferences such as "daily contact with relatives/close friends, usually attends church, temple, synagogue, etc." are also useful to activities care planning.

ACTIVITY CARE PLAN MODULE

The Activities Care Plan Module Committee[2] has developed care planning guidelines which reflect standards of practice for the activity professional (Department of Health and Human Services, in press). These guidelines were written to provide an overview of the philosophy of activities and crucial activity standards such as activity assessments. This Care Plan Module provides guidelines which can be applied to a variety of long term residents with multiple strengths and needs.

The December 1989 Draft of the Activities Care Plan Module (Cornelius et al., 1989) included an overview of activities. This overview described the relevance of activities to the lives of nursing home residents. It discussed basic concepts and definitions of activities, dynamics of activities and relevant risk factors, demographic characteristics associated with decline in activities, health related factors, skills and competence factors, and effects on quality of life.

2.The Activities Care Plan Module Committee was coordinated by the Health Care Financing Administration's resident assessment contractors.

The Module also contained information about trigger definitions, activities' preferences and history, care planning and adaptations, current status of resident needs, and follow-up guidelines. Several resources were listed at the end of the Module.

The MDS and the triggers are two areas of the resident assessment process which must be followed according to federal regulations; however, many of the other materials, i.e., care plan modules, are guidelines. The Activities Care Plan Module provides a direction for activity assessments and care planning, but it does not prescribe the exact route to be followed. This leaves open a door of flexibility which is necessary for individualized programming.

Each activity professional will need to continue developing activity assessment tools and effective care planning approaches. Activity professionals will be given some basic information about resident preferences from the MDS. More personalized information about preferences will be needed in order to complete a comprehensive assessment. If a resident indicates on the MDS a preference for music, the activity professional will need to interview this resident further to discuss the type of music the resident prefers, where and when the resident enjoys listening, whether the resident is a participant or listener in music, etc. (Perschbacher, 1989). This information will need to be documented in the resident's record, probably on an activity assessment form. The National Association of Activity Professionals has established standards of practice for activity professionals which can be used as a resource for establishing comprehensive activity assessments (National Association of Activity Professionals, 1989).

CONCLUSION

The mandated resident assessment provides a format for focusing on resident outcomes and the diversity and uniqueness of each nursing home resident. Recognition of the potential of this assessment tool will assure that Congress's desire for quality of life to become a part of daily nursing home life will be realized. Activity professionals will need to take an active role in this assessment process as it is implemented in October of 1990 and as it continues to be evaluated over the next few years. The focus of this assessment must remain on improving the lives of nursing home residents. Participating in this new challenge presents a felicitous opportunity to illustrate the impact of activities on positive resident outcomes.

REFERENCES

Cornelius, E., Cook, J., Perschbacher, R., Carlson, J., Hartman, M., Morris, A., Reublinger, V., Sinclair, S., and Wizik, E. (1989). Activities care plan module draft. Committee correspondence, December.

Department of Health and Human Services, Health Care Financing Administration (1989). Medicare and Medicaid; Requirements for long term care facilities; Final rule with request for comment. *Federal Register, 54* (21), p. 5316-5373.

Department of Health and Human Services (1989). *State operations manual: Provider certification* (Transmittal #232). Baltimore: Health Care Financing Administration.

Department of Health and Human Services (1990). Correspondence from Wayne Smith, Director of Office of Survey and Certification, to Associate Regional Administrators, Division of Health Standards and Quality, regarding Resident Assessment Instrument, April 30.

Department of Health and Human Services (in press). Activities care plan module: Developed under contract with the Health Care Financing Administration, contract no. 500-88-0055.

Institute of Medicine (1986). *Improving the quality of care in nursing homes.* Washington, D. C.: National Academy Press.

Morris, J. N., Hawes, C., Fries, B. E., Phillips, C. D., Mor, V., Katz, S., Murphy, K., Drugovich, M. L., and Friedlob, A. S. (1990). Designing the national resident assessment instrument for nursing homes. *The Gerontologist, 30* (3), 293-307.

National Association of Activity Professionals (1989). *Position on national certification for activity professionals.* Jackson, T., comp. Perschbacher, R., ed. Washington, DC: National Association of Activity Professionals.

Perschbacher, R. (1989). *Stepping forward with activities.* Asheville, NC: Bristlecone Consulting Company.

Leisure Activities
and Quality of Life

Letitia T. Jackson

There is a growing concern over the future of long term care in America. The growing number of elderly and disabled has created new roles for long term care facilities, such as nursing homes and residential care facilities, and facility personnel are expected to do more than provide basic nursing care. The traditional emphasis on quality of care has been joined by the new concern for quality of life. Consumers and health care professionals, especially long term care practitioners, agree that the nursing home should be a place for living to the fullest extent of an individual's capabilities (McDonald, 1982).

A life of high quality is difficult to define and even harder to measure. The concept of quality of life is very individual in nature, thus creating quite a challenge for long term care facilities. In a sense, quality of life for the elderly means involvement in stimulating, creative, and meaningful activity (Kane, 1987). McDonald, in a study commissioned by the American Health Care Association in 1982, has provided a definition of quality of life that has definite and positive implications for the recreation profession.

Letitia "Tish" T. Jackson is Coordinator of Project LIFE (Leisure Is For Everyone) in the Department of Parks, Recreation and Tourism at the University of Missouri-Columbia. She has 15 years experience as an activity professional, holds a Masters Degree in Recreation Administration and is certified as an Activity Consultant through the National Certification Council for Activity Professionals.

Ms. Jackson's presentation at the 1990 NAAP convention titled "Here's Proof: Activities Do Improve Quality of Life" was based upon this manuscript originally published in the Research Update section of *Parks & Recreation* (1988) April, Vol. 23, No. 4, pp. 19-24, 66. Reprinted by permission of *Parks & Recreation*, a magazine published by the National Recreation and Park Association, 12th Fl., 3101 Park Center Drive, Alexandria, VA 22302.

QUALITY OF LIFE DEFINED

McDonald's study presented a comprehensive approach to enhance the quality of life for residents in long term care facilities. Defining quality of life as a construct made up of several parts or components organized into six general categories, the resulting definition of quality of life can serve as the framework for individuals to build their own unique concept of quality of life. The first category in the definition is *Physical Wellbeing*. Components within it are material comforts, health and hygiene, and security. This category is largely met because of the large percentage of professionals involved in physical care giving and because mechanisms for reimbursement exist. *Interpersonal Relations* are the focus of the second category. This includes relationships with relatives, intimate relationships and community involvement. The third category is concerned with *Personal Development*. Components comprising this category are related to opportunities for intellectual development, self-expression, gainful activity and self-awareness. *Recreational Activities* are directly addressed as the fifth category in the McDonald definition of quality of life. This is further divided into three components: socializing, passive recreation and active recreation. The sixth and final category is *Spiritual and Transcendental Activities* involving self-understanding and symbolic activity as its components.

Activity professionals can use this emerging holistic concept of quality of life as a foundation for their accountability, their program philosophy and as justification in their role as a member of the interdisciplinary team. With an effective, well-planned program an activity professional can have an impact on each component of the quality of life of their residents. The remainder of this research review is illustrative, rather than exhaustive, citing research studies relating to leisure activities and their effects on some aspect of quality of life.

LAUGHTER IS GOOD MEDICINE

Adams and McGuire's (1986) study of elderly nursing home residents sought to determine the benefits of laughter by using humorous and non-humorous movies. The authors noticed that aged persons with long spans of idleness seemed to experience a greater degree of perceived pain. Idle persons have more time to dwell on their health problems and tend to become preoccupied with pain. They often get attention and reinforcement from others who are sympathetic to their complaint. Therefore, the researchers theorized that if the amount of unoccupied time were reduced then the degree of perceived pain would also decrease. Two basic hypotheses were tested and supported in this study. First, residents viewing humorous movies experienced a greater decrease in perceived pain than did residents viewing non-humorous movies. Second, residents viewing humorous movies experienced a greater improvement in affect than individuals viewing non-humorous movies. Affect was defined in this study as a global feeling toward present-day life. Members of the group viewing the humorous movies also required fewer PRN (as needed) medications than the other group during the course of the study. While this is important to activity professionals who are responsible for alleviating boredom in long term care facilities through the provision of creative and purposeful activity programs, it is also important for program planners working with non-institutionalized aged persons. Incorporating humor and laughter into a program should be a priority.

MUSIC AND VIDEO GAMES SHOWN EFFECTIVE

Wolfe (1983) investigated the effectiveness of a music-based group sensory training program in improving environmental awareness, activity participation level, reality orientation and attitude of regressed geriatric patients. The program consisted of activities combining the experiences of sound and music with other sensory stimuli. The sessions included identification of self and others, imitation and response, environmental awareness, auditory discrimination and awareness, breathing and relaxation, and identification of tactile, olfactory and gustatory stimuli. Recorded music, taped sounds, original music, percussion instruments and body instruments were used to facilitate interaction with and awareness of the environment. The author concluded that there were significant improvements in mental status scores, significant increases in sensory evaluation scores, significant changes in attitude scores, and significant increases in activity participation levels in the experimental group when compared to the control group. Results of this study also provide support for the belief that deterioration and regression are accelerated under conditions of isolation and stimulus deprivation.

Two separate studies concentrated on the effects of video games on long term care residents. The first examined the effectiveness of video games in improving the quality of life for residents in long term care facilities (McGuire, 1984). The author measured the self-esteem and affect of residents in an intermediate care facility who played video games during an eight week period. The video game group exhibited significant improvement in both self-esteem and affect from the pretest to the posttest. McGuire concluded that video games were effective in improving select attributes of quality of life for the residents who participated in the study and that the games offered unique stimulation and challenges.

Another related study investigated the impact of video games on the emotional states and affiliation behavior of nursing home residents (Riddick, Spector & Drogin, 1986). The findings of this study suggested that the arousal state of elderly residents could be affected by playing video games and that certain aspects of emotional well-being and affiliation behavior could be improved as well. The authors also noted that the video game program did not emerge as an effective method for improving the nursing home residents' pleasure and dominance states. The researchers suggested two possibly integrated explanations for this lack of improvement. It was possible that the participants did not feel sufficiently challenged by the games or that they did not perceive themselves to have mastered the skills necessary to play.

PHYSICAL ACTIVITIES CONTRIBUTE TO FEELINGS OF WELL-BEING

Activities affecting physical well-being range from active games and sports, dances, and exercises to movement therapy. Leitner and Leitner (1985) reported the physical benefits of exercise, such as increased comfort in movement and improvement in the performance of activities of daily living, as well as the mental benefits. They cited research which indicated that most individuals experienced a heightened sense of well-being after exercise. Exercise increased energy levels and served as an outlet for tension. The authors suggested that motivation to exercise can be increased if the leader created a recreational atmosphere, such as incorporating music into the sessions and using props (e.g., colorful scarves, funny hats, etc.).

Sandel (1987) reported several benefits of a movement therapy program initiated in a skilled nursing facility. Benefits included increases in self-expression, improved attitudes and willingness to exercise, increased interpersonal relationships and interest in assuming leadership roles in the group sessions.

SPIRITUALITY:
IMPORTANT BUT UNDERINVESTIGATED

The preceding research relates to one or more of the quality of life components identified by McDonald (1982). Although, it is well-known that activity directors in nursing homes coordinate bible study groups, church volunteer groups, and schedule the religious services in the facilities, the author of this research review did not find empirical research examining the spiritual quality of life in long term care facilities.

Cluff (1986), while stressing the importance of the spiritual and religious needs of older persons, especially those who are frail and disabled, cautions that sharing in the religious and spiritual concerns of an older person demands more than the fulfillment of tasks and deeds. Rather, it requires the investment and dedication of one's self in the life of another person. The author went further to state that a serious error today is making spirituality a problem to be resolved rather than an opportunity to be seized. Activity coordinators, in their holistic approach to programming activities, should take a serious look at the spiritual component of quality of life and evaluate whether or not the existing activity program is truly meeting the needs of their residents.

Each of these studies indicate a positive contribution of activities to the components that comprise quality of life. The evidence is accumulating but there remains an ever increasing need to conduct "outcome-related" research to expand the existing foundation of research documenting the importance of activities in long term care facilities.

REFERENCES

Adams, E., & McGuire, F. (1986). Is laughter the best medicine? A study of the effects of humor on perceived pain and affect. *Activities, Adaptation & Aging, 8* (3/4), 157-175.

Cluff, C. (1986). Spiritual intervention reconsidered. *Topics in Geriatric Rehabilitation, 1* (2), 77-82.

Kane, R. (1987). Quality of life in long-term institutions: Is a regulatory strategy feasible? *Danish Medical Bulletin,* (5), 73-81.

Leitner, M. & Leitner, S. (1985). *Leisure in later life.* New York: Haworth Press.

McDonald, T. (1982). *Target: Tomorrow.* Washington, D.C: American Health Care Association.

McGuire, F. (1984). Improving the quality of life for residents of long term care facilities through video games. *Activities, Adaptation & Aging, 6* (1), 1-7.

Riddick, C., Spector, S., & Drogin, E. (1986). The effects of videogame play on the emotional states and affiliative behavior of nursing home residents. *Activities, Adaptation & Aging, 8* (1), 95-107.

Sandel, S. & Johnson, D. (1987). *Waiting at the gate: Creativity and hope in the nursing home.* New York: Haworth Press.

Wolfe, J. (1983). The use of music in a group sensory training program for regressed geriatric patients. *Activities, Adaptation & Aging, 4* (1), 49-62.

Spirituality and Aging: Activity Key to "Holiest" Health Care

Diane S. Martin
Wendy G. Fuller

SUMMARY. A faith based discussion group can do much to enhance the quality of life of residents within the long term care setting. Each individual's spirituality is a link between self and others, past and present. The facilitator of such a group can use validation techniques and socio-therapeutic principles to lead members toward feelings of community wholeness, outwardly focused behavior and a renewed desire to contribute to society.

OPENING ADDRESS

Shalom — peace — friends and fellow travelers on life's exciting journey. We gather here in Seattle today to discuss the role activity professionals have in providing for the spiritual needs of the elderly whom we serve. We are here not to discuss a specific religious faith but to explore the facets of faith and the power they give our lives.

We are here to explore that huge mysterious force that "buoys us with ethical patterns and moves us with symbols and rituals."[1] Faith can be as different and unique as each of us in this room, yet we are one in our faith. On a very deep level, our faith has recognizably the same elements whether we are Christian or Jewish or Buddhist. There is an integrity in each person's honest faith that enlightens

Diane S. Martin, BFA in Art Education, ACC, is Director of the Activity Department at The Woodview, Long Term Care Facility, 103 Rosehill Drive, South Boston, VA 24592. Wendy G. Fuller, BA in Sociology, ACC, is the Expressive Arts Coordinator at The Woodview.

our own efforts to come close to the holy. We inform one another as, together, activity professionals seek the key to holiest health care for our adult and nursing home residents.

James Fowler, who expanded Erik Erikson's theory of life stages into a book, *The Stages of Faith*, says "faith is a coat against nakedness. Faith helps us form a dependable 'life space' — an ultimate environment. At a deeper level, faith undergirds us when our life space is punctured and collapses — when the felt reality of our ultimate environment proves to be less than ultimate."[2]

Consider these statements as we think about the environment of the institutional home. Its felt reality is certainly less than ultimate for those who live there. Our frail residents need their faith strengthened in order to form a new dependable life space.

Fowler also says, "Faith is a person's or group's way of moving into the force field of life."[3] For our residents, it is the way to move *back* into the force field of life when they think nursing home placement is the end of life.

Faith takes many forms. For our elderly residents faith, intertwined with the separate facets of religion and spirituality, forms the life ring that keeps them buoyed with ethical patterns and secured with symbol and ritual as they move back into the force field of life within the nursing home environment.

Edgar Mitchell, the astronaut, came back from the moon transformed by the spiritual experience he had in space. He said, "Religion is what we believe because someone else experienced it, while spirituality is what we believe because we have experienced it ourselves. The spiritual encounter is the one that transforms us and empowers us. So a spiritual approach will be the one in which the truth of one's experience is trusted."[4]

Holiest health care fosters health nurturing religion that keeps our residents connected to their religious tradition and to the truth of their spiritual roots, and lets them continue to trust in that truth. Holiest health care is person and creation centered. It provides residents with continued spiritual growth experiences in a climate of love.

Spirituality has to do with all of our connections in life. Spirituality is the link between past and present. It lifts us out and beyond our individual selves and links us with God and others and the universe. Spirituality is the only link between mind and body. Holiest health care seeks to strengthen this link and these connections by offering another way to look at the world — through a spiritual lens. Through this spirit lens one can begin to move from victim and anger to that inner peace out of which healing takes place. Healing; the word's Greek roots say it all. Heal, holy, hale (and hearty) and whole are root words. To *not* be whole is to be broken. To be broken is to be in spiritual distress.

How do we identify who among our residents is in spiritual distress? Three cues are: helplessness, hopelessness and withdrawal. These residents may exhibit emotional deadness or they may appear suspicious. They may hang onto worn out behavior patterns such as blaming. Others may be physically or verbally withdrawn and refuse to be intimate with anyone. They have lost the ability to love; most of all to love themselves.

Fox, in his book *The Coming of the Cosmic Christ*, says, "Self love is a rare and radical kind of love because it requires a trust of our right to be here and of the universe's love of us."[5]

How many of those we try to reach have no trust of their right to be here; to be still alive! Perhaps they feel it is the unspoken message from families who have "relegated" them to the institution. They feel forsaken. Their value and worth as human beings is threatened and perhaps even negated as the world goes busily by. They feel cut off from loved ones and this feeling of alienation often extends into feelings about their relationship with God.

The only way they will begin to regain that love of themselves, and to trust their right to be alive, is by experiencing God's unconditional love through people; through you and me. We must love our residents through total acceptance of them as they are.

This charge seems overwhelming in the face of the reality and vastness of our job description. Yet we are where we are most of all to love. We are not hired to judge or even to counsel people, though we assess and write progress notes. We are therapists, even though we do not claim our rightful title. Therapy means to interact with a divinity or human being. We interact daily and are uniquely placed to give unconditional love to our residents in both the individual and group setting.

To give this kind of love, we have to be very good listeners and watchers. We have to tune into messages sent through body language, looks and unspoken words. We have to wait, sometimes a long time, to be invited into a resident's life.

Then there are those other residents who give their call for help and for love by slipping away from the unendurable present to the safety of the past. For no apparent organic reason, they become disoriented. Their spiritual connections are broken. Yet we can help them also through our love as we affirm them in whatever stage of orientation they are. We can validate them for whom they perceive themselves to be as we work to build their trust.

The "sundowner" who must fix dinner every evening at five can be affirmed as a good wife and mother who is concerned for the welfare of her family. *Validation, The Feil Method* by Naomi Feil, is an invaluable book on the subject of affirmation. This type of sensitive response will help in the building of trust. Those of us who work with the elderly know there is no one formula since each person is different. Each of us will have to discover within ourselves the way to empathize with the disoriented elderly.

This trust building—one on one—is the vital key to drawing residents into small groups where continued love and socio-therapeutic skills can be used to promote spiritual growth and healing. Ultimately it is within a loving community that wholeness takes place. It is in the group that we can provide integrating, energizing, growing relationships with that loving spirit religions call God.

The Woodview Bible study group is just such a group and it has been challenged by disoriented and maloriented residents. One such resident, who was maloriented, burdened every small group conversation with her daily litany of losses. With the leader's and group's help, today she is able to count her blessings.

Community groups that provide health nurturing religious experiences for the "old old" should be multifaceted. When we interact with those who have organic brain disease, strokes and other mental illnesses, we need to remember parts of the brain, controlling specific responses, may be damaged.

The left side of the brain operates the motor function of the right side of our body, while the right brain operates motor functions of the left side. We need to provide experiences that speak to both sides of the brain, both logical and intuitive, that will even possibly help with the reintegration process.

In this vein, I introduce one last major theory. It is a theory to which I was introduced in Dr. Howard Clinebell's continuing education program for clergy at Virginia Theological Seminary around 1979. It is his theory of whole brain religion. Like most theories, it is complex and not fully proven and, like most theories, it can be used with "playful seriousness and serious playfulness."[6] The theory, however, defines and illumines what we have been doing and the responses we get in our religious activity therapies.

Clinebell notes whole brain religion as having characteristic left and right brain functions. Doing, works, seriousness and loving God with one's mind are left brain functions. Correspondingly, on the right side one experiences being, grace, playfulness and religious experiences such as meditation and communion. Basically the left represents masculine characteristics and the right represents feminine qualities.[7]

Keep this division in mind as I share a short composite of some of the activities we have designed for our residents who are Bible Belt stalwarts. We leaders also reflect the Christian faith in our life and work.

We are not baptized in lemon juice! Being a Christian is joyous and fun when one explores the Word through clowning and dancing and singing. Writing and painting also extend ones experience of the holy. Both great and small revelations come from the creative activity.

Visual art activities stretch imaginations toward the heavens. Psalm 104 can speak to the soul of those with organic brain disease. One such resident, even though nearly blind and deaf, spent an hour expressing the Psalm's message with great intuitive clarity. Her penciled drawing was worthy of the mystical artist, William Blake.

In Library Club, residents compose group poems that recreate their sense of belonging to a beautiful earth. In Bible study, residents write their own psalms of lament, faith and praise. They dance the Lord's Prayer in shared communion.

Music speaks to those with Alzheimer's, to the withdrawn, and to the alert. Our residents sing, almost daily, their hymns of praise, never forgetting the words and learning many new ones. They use their songs of faith not only to enrich their own souls but to reach out to roombound neighbors.

These are all right brain activities. They have to do with our heart level conviction, with timelessness and eternity. The right side celebrates the mystery of life while acknowledging God's protective cloak around us. The right side of our brain responds in a heartfelt way when reasoning powers are diminished or gone.

On the left side of whole brain religion we have duty, our belief system, and our ethics. The last segment of this workshop will show how Bible study groups or other faith groups can use these left brain religion functions to build a sense of renewed self-worth in residents and finally a greater sense of community within the nursing home. Only within community can wholeness occur.

Bible study lets residents remember their beginnings, the foundations of their faith. Through recalling past experiences, they remember the simple but profound truth that they have been carried successfully through life on the strong shoulders of faith. They are reminded of God's great love for them as they share their stories.

Bible study also reminds residents of their ethics, the codes they lived by and need to pull out now to survive in a less than ultimate environment. It reminds them of their responsibilities and helps them crawl out of their cocoons to reach out in caring to those who work and live and die within the home. It makes them want to reach out further to contribute to the community outside the home as it connects them to the greater world.

With all of this spiritual activity comes a renewed sense of self-worth, a re-birth of self love and even often a return from disorientation or malorientation. Unconditionally loved, stimulated with opportunities for experiencing spiritual growth through Bible study and expressive arts modalities in a community of faith, healing truly takes place for our residents.

This we believe is the activity key to holiest health care.

PARTICIPATORY SESSION

At this point, the group of 110 activity directors was asked the following three questions in preparation for a discussion on facilitating a faith group:

1. What would you like to see in your facility? Describe "utopia," the perfect nursing home.
2. What barriers exist that keep us from reaching "utopia"?
3. What strengths do our residents have at this point in their lives?

Their responses follow:

Utopia

normalcy	laughter	future oriented activities
smiles	touching	goal oriented activities
conversation	hugs	community spirit
private space	friendliness	animals/children/visitors
live plants	cleanliness	residents getting outdoors
residents making music	volunteers	resident helping resident
lots of "happy stuff"	residents eager to get involved	

Barriers

loss of self esteem	loss of identity
loss of body parts & functions	loss of friends/family
loss of decision making/choice	loss of dignity
loss of possessions	social hierarchy
loss of privacy	prejudice-racial/cultural
learned helplessness	loss of memory
loss of pets and home cooking	feeling of no longer being a productive member of society

Strengths

they are survivors	ability to learn
lifetime of experience	wisdom
faith	special talents
sense of humor	acceptance
have loved	tolerance/patience in some areas
have been loved	creativity
leadership qualities	intelligence
emotional support from family/friends	

PURPOSE

The purpose of a Bible study group, or faith group, is to utilize residents strengths that break through these barriers. The goal is to reach a state of "utopia" or good, solid community spirit among residents and staff.

At The Woodview long term care facility, in South Boston, Virginia, such a group has existed for four years with positive changes noted. Residents are more tolerant of one another and more patient with themselves and staff. Self esteem and self confidence are improved, intellects are challenged and new skills learned. Residents, given the opportunity to contribute successfully to nursing home life, respond positively. They support each other, focusing outwardly rather than inwardly. They take an interest in helping others, both in and outside the facility.

WHO LEADS THE GROUP

The leader of a Jewish or Christian faith group need not be a biblical scholar, but a facilitator adept at getting the group members talking and keeping them talking, as well as listening, learning and contributing. The leader understands that each individual can contribute, no matter what his level of orientation to reality. The group leader can be a staff member, chaplain, or a volunteer. The leader's most important qualification is knowing each group member, and earning his trust. This takes time. It involves much one to one interaction and, until that trust develops, there is little chance that the group will function as it should. At The Woodview, the group facilitator is a member of the activity department. This has enabled her to work closely with the residents on a day to day basis; to observe their interaction with others in their daily life, and to share both successes and frustrations. In many cases she knows the resident's children, grandchildren, and great-grandchildren. Group leader and group member are friends, each respecting the other's feelings and moods; each believing in the other. Only among trusted friends can true sharing take place and growth be initiated.

WHO PARTICIPATES IN THE GROUP

Members should be mobile enough to be transported to the meeting room.
A faith group will most likely be comprised of residents at varying levels of orientation; indeed, this should be encouraged. At The Woodview, maloriented residents benefit from such a group. They add a special dimension and are an interesting challenge to leader and members alike. Alert, oriented residents will be the backbone of the group in the beginning, but confused, non-verbal, and aphasic residents can also add much and should be included. Extremely disruptive residents should not be included. This is not to say that disruptive residents have no spiritual needs, but rather that those needs should be met in other ways. Group attendance is, of course, strictly voluntary with the size determined by space available and the leader's judgement. The Woodview finds 30 an effectively workable group.

A MODEL GROUP

Structure is important to the elderly. Routine means comfort, so, at The Woodview, the same format for the one hour long meeting is used each week.

I. *Welcome and Affirmation* that there is work to be done. (i.e., this is not entertainment. This is a group with a purpose.)

II. *Opening Prayer* including prayers of intercession. The opening prayer always offers thanks for the opportunity to meet together as a group, asks for love, patience, etc. and asks special help for those in need. This list of "prayer requests" is obtained from the group and may include other residents, families, friends, staff members, government leaders, or even a prayer for oneself.

III. *Sharing Time.* Frequently, group members will bring with them a favorite poem, scripture verse or magazine article. This is read and discussed by the group.

IV. *Lesson/Discussion.* This need not be from the Bible. Spirituality is found all around us. Literature offers an endless supply of appropriate material. Even some comic strips work. The point is that the lesson focus on the needs/desires of the group. The group leader presents the material, asks a leading question, and lets the conversational interchange begin. The facilitator should take care not to be over prepared with theological background information. Her/his role is to get the group talking, not to give a sermon!

V. *Closing Prayer.* At The Woodview, the group has chosen to close each session by saying "The Lord's Prayer" together. (In recent months, it has been "dancing" the prayer.)

VI. *Final Affirmation.* The group is thanked for coming and the leader shares her enjoyment of the session and the contributions of the participants.

VII. *Post-Group Discussions.* This is essential for residents who are hesitant to speak in groups. Many residents have never spoken up, and never will speak up, but, given the opportunity in a one to one setting, will pour forth a plethora of comments, ideas, and feelings. It is the responsibility of the group leader to target these residents each week, immediately after the session, for private conversation. Appropriate suggestions/comments can then be shared at the next group meeting, giving credit to the originator. Thus, even the shy are making contributions.

SAMPLE LESSONS FOR DISCUSSION

(Note: These are two of the 20 lessons studied by small groups during the NAAP '90 Workshop. The following discussion questions were written by the participants in Seattle. They were given 10 minutes to prepare the questions.)

I. Psalm 71, from *The Bible* (see *Good News or RSV*). This Psalm is known as a "Prayer For Help in Old Age."

Discussion Questions

1. Consider the first three verses. What is this passage about?
2. What lessons can we learn from it?
3. How can we apply it to our lives?
4. To whom do we go for help?
5. Who or what do we turn to when we are confused?
6. Do we ever feel that God is silent?
7. What makes you know that God is listening to you?

II. THAT'S WHY I'M A VERY REMARKABLE FELLOW
William L. Stidger

"Seventh Heaven" is one of the truly great movies. If you ever get a chance to see it, don't miss it! It was first released many years ago as a silent picture and later with sound. One of the most unforgettable scenes in the story pictures Chico, who is the hero of the story, and the rat down in the dirty sewers beneath the streets of Paris. Chico works there. Suddenly a great gush of water poured from a manhole above and swept the rat into the river of vile smelling sewage. The rat might have drowned had not Chico unloaded some of his wholesome philosophy of life as he said, "I work in the sewers, Rat, but I live in the stars." Then he gave the rat some good advice: "Never look down! Always look up! I never look down!! I always look up! That's why I'm a very remarkable fellow."

The rat cocked his head and listened carefully as though he understood every word. After all, wasn't Chico a very important person? Hadn't he just saved him from almost certain death? Chico continued his lecture and concluded with the words: "For those who will climb it, Rat, there is a ladder which leads from the sewer to the stars! And as you climb, Fellow, keep looking up! I always look up! I never look down! That's why I'm a very remarkable fellow!"

Chico's philosophy worked for him, as it will work for us. As the story continues, he climbed from the sewer to the street level of life; and then to a life of love, which was Seventh Heaven. I think that all of us have a bit of Chico in us. Maybe he was echoing something the Psalmist said many years ago in Psalm 121:11, "I lift up my eyes." Keep looking up!

Adapted from *There Are Sermons in Stories*, by William L. Stidger.[8]

Discussion Questions

1. Have you ever been rescued?
2. Have you ever been like the rat and needed rescuing?
3. Have you ever been like Chico and rescued someone else?

4. Right now, is there someone in your life that you could give some help to and rescue?

OUTGROWTH FROM THE GROUP

It is important for group members to have a purpose, even beyond the obvious opportunities to talk, learn and improve interpersonal relationships. At The Woodview, some interesting outgrowths have occurred. The group has learned to write prayers, sermons and psalms which have been "published" in the facility newsletter, used in special services at the home and even read at churches in the community. The group has written, rehearsed and performed special devotional services and Christmas pageants. The group has also taken as its responsibility the writing of the memorial remembrances that are used in services at the home. All of these have enhanced the group's feelings of successfully contributing to society, and affirmed feelings of self-worth.

CONCLUSION

In the four years since The Woodview's Bible study group began, many positive changes occurred. A slow process, with "utopia" still an activity director's dream, perhaps the most obvious change has been the group itself. With intellect challenged, the group has matured. Discussions have become noticeably more detailed and deep. Residents now readily open up and reach out to each other to work through problems. Abstract thinking is evident in residents who were once mono-syllabic. Residents, who once saw only the negatives in their lives, are now able to look at the positives and count their blessings. The group has learned to affirm and accept both self and others.

Outside the group these new strengths and feelings carry over. Group members become friends and seek each other's company. Mobile residents take an interest in visiting those who can't get out. There is evidence of resident helping resident during other activities and throughout the day. They are more tolerant of one another's differences.

Perhaps the most exciting change is that residents are eager and willing to learn new things! Their fear has been lessened while self-confidence and a desire to help others has been restored. We observe that the residents have been spiritually revitalized, gone on to create a sense of community within The Woodview; evidence that the spiritual approach is the key to Holiest Health Care.

NOTES

1. James Fowler, *Stages of Faith, The Psychology of Human Development and the Quest for Meaning*, San Francisco, CA, Harper and Row, 1981, pp. xxiii.
2. Ibid, pp. xii.
3. Ibid., pp. 4.
4. Lois B. Robbins, *Waking Up In the Age of Creativity*, Santa Fe, New Mexico, Bear and Co., 1985. pp. 18.
5. Matthew Fox, *The Coming of the Cosmic Christ*, San Francisco, CA, Harper and Row, 1988, pp. 21.
6. James Fowler, *Stages of Faith, The Psychology of Human Development and the Quest for Meaning*, San Francisco, CA, Harper and Row, 1981, pp. vii, quoting Erik Erikson.
7. Concept explored by Howard Clinebell, *Contemporary Growth Therapies*, Nashville, TN, Abingdon Press, 1981.
8. "That's Why I'm a Very Remarkable Fellow" by William L. Stidger from *34 Two-Minute Talks*, Stanley P. Cornils, Editor. Standard Publishing Co.; Cincinnati, Ohio, 1985.

BIBLIOGRAPHY

Clinebell, Howard, *Contemporary Growth Therapies*, Abingdon Press, Nashville, TN 1981.

Cornils, Stanley P., *34 Two-Minute Talks*, Standard Publishing Co., Cincinnati, Ohio, 1985.

Feil, Naomi ASCW *Validation, The Feil Method*, Edward Feil Productions, Cleveland, Ohio, 1988.

Fowler, James W., *Stages of Faith, The Psychology of Human Development and the Quest for Meaning*, Harper and Row, San Francisco, CA, 1981.

Fox, Matthew, *The Coming of the Cosmic Christ*, Harper and Row, San Francisco, CA, 1988.

Gibran, Kahil, *The Prophet*, Alfred A. Knopf, Inc., New York, 1923.

Peck, Carol F., *From Deep Within*, The Haworth Press, New York, 1989.

Robbins, Lois B., *Waking Up in the Age of Creativity*, Bear and Co., Santa Fe, NM, 1985.

Short, Robert, *The Gospel According to Peanuts*, John Knox Press, Richmond, VA, 1964.

Weiss, Jules C., *Expressive Therapy with Elders and the Disabled, Touching the Heart of Life*, The Haworth Press, New York, London, 1984.

Woods, Robert, *Symbion*, Bear & Company, Inc., Sante Fe, New Mexico, 1982.

Affirmative Aging — A Resource for Ministry, The Episcopal Society for Ministry in Aging, 1985.

The New National Baptist Hymnal, National Baptist Publishing Board, Nashville, TN 1977.

Good News Bible, 1976.

Holy Bible, Revised Standard Version, 1952.

Relocation and the Resident

Joan T. Harkulich
Christine Brugler

SUMMARY. Relocation of a chronically ill aged client causes relocation stress, and staff working in long term care facilities need to interact and plan care in such a manner as to reduce problems associated with this relocation. The authors discuss territoriality and its interrelationship with relocation, as well as the types of relocation that the aged client might experience. Staff working in long term care facilities should be helped by learning which client is most at risk for relocation stress, the procedure to use when relocation must happen, monitoring of the relocated client, plans for the relocated client and some suggestions to use when the client must leave the facility.

A PLACE TO CALL MY VERY OWN

Space, and the objects occupying the space, are very important. If you think about your home, you probably have a favorite easy chair that you like to relax on after a busy day, a certain seating arrangement around the dinner table, or even a special picture or artwork that may hang on your wall. In all of these instances, you have control and choice. For example, you could have chosen the

Joan T. Harkulich and Christine Brugler both received their MSN degrees at Kent State University and work in the area of long term care. Christine is a consultant at Hillside Hospital in Warren, OH and Joan is the Director of Research and Professional Services at Care Services, Beachwood, OH, which is a corporation that owns six nursing homes. They have just completed a study to validate the Nursing diagnosis of "Translocation Syndrome."

The research for this study was partially funded by the Peg Schlitz Fund of Delta Xi Chapter of Sigma Theta Tau (at Kent State University).

Correspondence should be addressed to Joan T. Harkulich, 3601 S. Green Road, Beachwood, OH 44122.

51

sofa instead of the chair as your favorite spot, you could change the seating arrangement around your dinner table whenever you choose, and if you do not like the artwork on one wall, you could change walls. Your need for, and control of space is great.

TERRITORIALITY – THE STUDY OF SPACE

The study of our behavior in space, or territoriality, was first researched in the animal kingdom. Hall (1966) defines territoriality as the behavior by which an organism lays claim to an area and defends it against members of its own species. We have heard how the lion of the jungle will fight off other animals, even other lions, who enter his territory. Most household pets will bark and be very cautious when strangers enter their territories.

Just like other animals, we are very protective of our territories. We may not fight with another adult who chooses to sit in our easy chair, but we might be uncomfortable or even reluctant to let the adult sit there. Children will often be very territorial, using the phrases "It's mine," or "I had it first," when they play. All people of all ages need some space, some territory to call their own.

Now, why do we all behave in this manner? Researchers debate whether territoriality is culturally learned, or just part of our make-up (genetically determined). Hall (1966) suggested that not only is territoriality part of our individual make-up but that it is just as important to us as food, water or air.

Perhaps you never thought of space, and your control of space as being that important. According to many researchers, in a crowded situation, new norms of behavior evolve, which are basically those of noninvolvement. It is easier to envision the importance of space when we don't have choices or control of a situation. Think of a time when your control of space was very limited, for instance in a crowded elevator. Because of the restricted physical control, you will often adapt psychologically. You restrain your eye contact, rarely looking at other people in the elevator, but at the numbers indicating the floors that the elevator has or will approach. Your conversation is greatly reduced, even if you were talking with a friend before getting into the elevator.

We now know that we are all territorial, but what do we gain by it? Ardrey (1966) suggests that humans strive to acquire and defend territory because it provides us with a sense of identity, stimulation, and security. Let's look at each of these issues.

Identity — The physical space we claim often becomes a reflection of ourselves. Our homes are decorated according to our likes and interests, whether that decor is country, modern or a little bit of everything. Having a space to call our own also yields an opportunity for self-expression. Perhaps at our work territory, we need to dress a certain way to express professionalism, but upon returning home, we can express our true selves wearing jeans and sneakers.

Stimulation — Where are you when your best ideas come to you? Chances are, you are in your own territory, whether at home, work, or in your car. For example, when you were in school, you had a favorite place to study, be it the library, your room, or at a friend's house. Studying became most productive and stimulating in a certain area of your territory.

Security — When we are at a place where we have control, we will feel more at ease, and less threatened. We feel more secure at our own homes, our own offices, our own cars, and our other territories than we do elsewhere.

TERRITORIALITY
AND THE NURSING HOME RESIDENT

All individuals' need for space, along with the control and use of it, is very important. This is especially true in the nursing home setting, where the residents' identity, stimulation, and feeling of security is vital for contentment and happiness. The residents' rooms become their personal territories, and along with their belongings, are most significant, a sweater . . . the smell of a certain perfume . . . a treasured photo . . . mean so much to some residents. Other residents, family members, and health-care workers need to be aware of territoriality concerns as they relate to institutionalized members of society.

RELOCATION

Relocation (translocation) refers to the movement of an individual from one place or environment to another. Much research has centered on relocation and some authors (Gordon, 1985; Brugler, 1986) refer to the untoward effects of the move as "translocation syndrome."

Relocation is stressful for people of all ages, but might especially affect elderly persons moving to a more restrictive environment. Borup (1982) suggested that older persons may experience four types of environmental relocation: residential, inter-institutional, intra-institutional, and residential/institutional. A brief discussion of these types of relocations will follow.

Residential — This move, from one residence to another, often is the least stressful of the four mentioned moves. If an individual decides to move from his/her home or apartment to another living dwelling, it is often by choice. The individual will often have control, for instance, deciding the location, amount of space, and decor of the new home. Usually the more decision making skills and control that is involved in the move, the less stressful the move becomes.

Inter-institutional — This move is between institutions, for example, from a hospital to a nursing home, from a nursing home to a hospital, or from one nursing home to another nursing home.

Intra-institutional — This is movement within the institution (nursing home or hospital). It could be from one unit to another, one room to another, or one floor to another. Reasons for this type of relocation could include: the need for the resident to move to a unit with a different acuity level; or a resident chooses a different room to move away from personal annoyances (a noisy or talkative roommate, a distracting window view, the sound of an ice machine, etc.).

Residential/Institutional — This move refers to the individual moving from his/her home to a hospital or nursing home. Admittance to a hospital is usually less stressful than the nursing home. If all factors are equal, a hospital stay is usually a short term stay as opposed to that of the nursing home which might be a permanent stay.

Elderly persons may be subjected to one or more of the above moves. The two factors of control and choice play very important roles in determining the residents' adaptation to the relocation.

PROCEDURE FOR RELOCATION

As stated before, many residents elect to move to another location in the nursing home. Sometimes the nursing home staff must relocate residents because they no longer need a distinct part of the facility, or their condition changes and they may need to be moved to receive more individualized care. Roommates go to the hospital or die, and staff want to move the remaining residents to an area which will enable staff to support and help them cope with the loss. Finally, sometimes either residents or families request a move.

Nursing homes strive to keep relocation to a minimum. However, if relocation within the facility must be done, the procedure outlined below will help make this move as painless as possible.

Procedure

1. All moves will be decided by a team of staff members, not by one individual.
2. Whenever possible, the resident will be involved in the decision to make the move.
3. Whenever possible, family members will be included in the decision to make the move.
4. Whenever possible, a room will be chosen to match the existing room (same bed location, same view, same area, same environmental outlay, etc.).
5. The resident will be taken to the new location and shown the new areas prior to the move.
6. The resident will be allowed to eat or join in other activities on the new unit, prior to the move.
7. On moving day, the resident will be permitted to move personal items and place them in the new room.
8. On moving day, family members will be encouraged to join the resident and help him/her move.

9. Whenever possible a staff member who is well-liked by the resident will help in the move.
10. On moving day the resident will be closely monitored by the staff on the new unit.
11. After the move, staff from the previous unit will be encouraged to visit the resident, so that there is no feeling of abandonment.
12. After the move, the new staff will be encouraged to contact the other staff for information, sharing of techniques, etc. to insure a continuity of care.
13. The prior roommate of the relocated resident will also be supported by the staff so that the roommate does not feel responsible for the move, feel guilty or abandoned.
14. If the old roommate desires to visit on the new unit, staff will help with this visit.

MONITORING OF RELOCATED RESIDENTS

Once the resident has been relocated to another room or when a resident is a new admission to the nursing home, staff may carefully monitor the resident for the behaviors shown on Table 1.

The staff may also monitor any positive statements made by the resident or any increase in socialization, weight and appetite increases, more positive attitude portrayed, increase in attendance at activities, and increases in involvement with other residents. Family members will be advised of any behaviors either positive or negative which staff members observe.

PLANS

If any resident suffers from relocation stress, staff may develop an individualized plan to assist the resident. Many therapies may be used, because each resident is unique and needs a specific intervention. It should be understood by the resident and family that an additional move might at times be the intervention of choice.

Some interventions included in the plan of care might be to:

TABLE 1

BEHAVIOR	PRESENT	ABSENT	PLAN
loneliness			
apprehension			
depression			
anxiety			
demonstration of insecurity in new living situation			
change in sleep patterns			
increased verbalization of needs			
change in eating habits			
verbalization of insecurity in new living situation			
weight change			
withdrawal			
demonstration of dependency			
demonstration of lack of trust			
verbalization of lack of trust in the staff			
verbalization of dependency			

(Harkulich, Brugler (1989))

1. Offer choices of space, room arrangement, and decorations.
2. Offer special foods to encourage the resident to eat.
3. Ask another resident to befriend the translocated resident.
4. Allow resident to visit friends and staff on old unit.
5. Point out the positives to the resident because of the move.
6. Hug/touch therapy by the new staff.
7. Reassurance by all staff and especially night staff.

8. Use warm milk, backrubs, white noise, etc. to insure an adequate night's sleep.
9. Communicate with family members regarding the adjustment of the resident as well as the family's role in helping the resident adjust.
10. Answer lights and questions as promptly as possible.
11. Encourage involvement in activities.
12. Encourage the resident to eat meals with other residents.
13. One-on-one visits by activity or social worker staff.
14. *_____
15. *_____
16. *_____
   *suggestions from families or staff

RELOCATION TO ANOTHER FACILITY

When residents live in a nursing home for a time, a bond develops between the residents and the staff and relocation to another institution (hospital, supportive housing or another nursing home) might be traumatic. For staff and residents alike, the relocation might be termed "a loss of a family member." Sometimes the relocation must be done and staff will be encouraged to help the residents as much as possible.

The following interventions might help these residents:

1. Reassure the residents that they will be able to return to the nursing home (if at all possible).
2. Have staff or other residents send cards to residents.
3. Visit residents if possible in the new location.
4. Phone families to check on the condition of the residents.
5. Hold residents' hands on the way out of facility into the ambulance if at all possible, or accompany them to the new facility.
6. Make sure residents have eye glasses, teeth, hearing aid, etc. close at hand if needed. Make sure head is covered, and not exposed to the elements.
7. Communicate to residents that staff at the nursing home care

about the residents and have no intention of abandoning them.

8. Communicate to residents that priest, rabbi or minister will be notified of the transfer.
9. Prepare residents as much as possible for the move using TENDER LOVING CARE in words and actions.
10. Communicate to residents that you will think about them. Let them know that they will not be out of sight/out of mind.
11. *_____
12. *_____
    * suggestions from family or staff

RESIDENTS AT RISK TO SUFFER FROM RELOCATION STRESS

Many residents in long term care facilities are at high risk for relocation stress. When considering losses previously suffered, coupled with many crises in their lives, the following residents might be considered at high risk for this stress:

1. Acutely or chronically ill residents
2. Depressed or anxious residents
3. Demented residents
4. Those who recently relocated from home, hospital or another facility
5. Those who enjoy ruts and hate to abandon them
6. Withdrawn residents and those who deny existence of any problems
7. Residents with a low self-esteem and those dissatisfied with life
8. Residents with little family support
9. Residents who are blind and need to memorize a new location

CONCLUSION

Relocation of nursing home residents is a stressful event. Whether residents are first admitted to a nursing home, moving from one nursing home to another, or moving to a different room within the same facility, the process involves the re-establishing of personal territories and bonds. Being aware of the significance of territoriality, namely the use of and control of space, is important to insure a smooth transition and decrease any untoward reactions to the move.

REFERENCES

Ardrey, R. (1966). *The territorial imperative: A personal inquiry into the animal origins of property and nations.* 1st.Ed. New York: Anthenum Press.

Borup, J.H. (1982). The effects of varying degrees of interinstitutional environmental change on long-term care patients. *The Gerontologist.* 22 (41), 405-417.

Brooke, V. (1989). How elders adjust. *Geriatric Nursing.* Mar/Apr. 66-68.

Brugler, C. (1986). *The defining characteristics of translocation syndrome – A validation study.* Unpublished paper. Kent State University.

Gordon, M. (1985). *Manual of nursing diagnosis.* New York: McGraw-Hill Book Co. p.214.

Hall, E. T. (1966). *The hidden dimension.* New York: Doubleday and Co.

Harkulich, J. & Brugler, C. (1989). Nursing Diagnosis/Translocation syndrome: Expert validation study. *People to People Journal.*

Harkulich, J. & Brugler, C. (1989). *Relocation and the resident: Information for family and friends.* Beachwood, Ohio: Care Services.

BIBLIOGRAPHY

Amenta, M., Weiner, A. & Amenta, D. (1984). Successful relocation of elderly residents. *Geriatric Nursing.* Nov/Dec., 356-360.

Brown, M., Cornwell, J. & Weist, J. (1981). Reducing the risks to the institutionalized elderly. *Journal of Gerontological Nursing.* 7 (7), 401-403.

Brand, F. & Smith, R. (1974). Life adjustment and relocation of the elderly. *Journal of Gerontology.* 29 (3), 336-340.

Chenita, W.C. (1983). Entry into a nursing home as a status passage: A theory to guide nursing practice. *Geriatric Nursing.* March/April, 92-97.

Engle, V. (1985). Temporary relocation: Is it stressful to your patients? *Journal of Gerontological Nursing.* 11 (10), 28-31.

Lange, J.L. (1980). Voluntary relocation among the elderly: Nursing implications. *Journal of Gerontological Nursing.* 6 (3), 405-407.

Rosswurm, M.A. (1983). Relocation and the elderly. *Journal of Gerontological Nursing.* 6 (12), 632-637.

Wolanin, M.O. (1978). Relocation of the elderly. *Journal of Gerontological Nursing.* 4 (3), 47-50.

Functioning as a Department Head and Supervisor: A New Role for the Activity Coordinator

Kathleen J. Halberg
Ellen Waters

SUMMARY. Although activity programs have grown significantly more sophisticated during their relatively short history, recognition and acceptance of their importance lags behind these advances. The major reason for this may be that many activity coordinators continue to function primarily as activity leaders rather than department heads and supervisors. This article presents basic information about how to employ and supervise activity assistants and work effectively with other staff. Employing (job descriptions, interviewing, and selecting), orienting and training, motivating, and evaluating activity assistants are reviewed, and orienting and gaining the cooperation of other staff, especially nursing staff, are discussed.

Many activity coordinators continually face the problem of lack of recognition of the importance of their programs by administrators and other staff. This may be the result of the activity coordinator not functioning primarily as a department head and supervisor. If current activity programs are to truly actualize their potential to play a major part in residents continuing to experience living in a meaningful and satisfying manner, a change in the role of the activity coordinator is needed. The purposes of this article are to discuss the

Kathleen J. Halberg is Associate Professor in the Department of Recreation and Leisure Studies at California State University, Long Beach, 1250 Bellflower Boulevard, Long Beach, CA 90840. Ellen Waters is Activity Coordinator at Ivorena Care Center, 687 Cheshire, Eugene, OR 97402.

importance of the activities coordinator functioning as a department head and supervisor, provide an overview of employing and supervising activity assistants, and review working effectively with other staff from the perspective of a department head.

FUNCTIONING AS A DEPARTMENT HEAD AND SUPERVISOR

The need for activity coordinators to begin to function more as department heads and supervisors is apparent in discussions with numerous activity professionals who frequently express a variety of problems with employing and retaining activity assistants and working effectively with other staff. Common complaints about activity assistants include depending on them to meet their responsibilities and meeting their duties at an acceptable level. Frequent absences from work and high turnover are problems as well. Gaining the acceptance and assistance of other staff, especially nursing staff, is a chronic problem and one of the most frequent complaints of activity coordinators.

High Turnover: A Reality with Activity Assistants

While the reasons for these commonly expressed problems undoubtedly vary, they appear to be based upon two basic issues. First, because of low salaries and other employment possibilities, retention of appropriate activity assistants is genuinely difficult. Since job turnover among activity coordinators is rather common, promotion from the assistant's to the coordinator's role is a frequent occurrence. It is to be expected and entirely reasonable that they will seek higher paying positions which provide greater responsibility and autonomy. Activity coordinators may just have to accept the fact that competent activity assistants will move on to better jobs, provide them with the best training and supervision possible, and wish them well in their new positions. From the broader perspective of the activity profession, however, thoroughly orienting and training new practitioners at the entry level as activity assistants will result in the continued upgrading of the profession.

Developing a Self-Image
as a Department Head

The second reason for these problems, both with activity assistants and other staff, may well be that the roles of supervisor and department head are relatively new to many activity coordinators. Many have little experience with and may be uncomfortable with these new roles.

Perhaps the most important step in becoming more comfortable with functioning as a department head and supervisor is that activity coordinators need to move beyond a view of themselves as staff members who primarily lead activities with residents. This step may not be easy for many activity coordinators since they most likely originally assumed their positions because they wanted to work directly with residents, became very effective in that role, and gained satisfaction through doing their jobs well and leading resident activities. While directly leading activities is the core of the activity program, activity coordinators must begin to think of themselves as department heads if the program is to receive the recognition it deserves.

To truly actualized the potential of the activity program, coordinators must learn to use their considerable talents to reach the greatest number of residents possible. The way to use these talents most efficiently is through supervising and managing activity assistants, other staff, and volunteers so that they are able to effectively work directly with residents. Even though most activity coordinators have a great deal of energy and frequently work long days and weeks, there simply are not enough hours in a day or a week to function both as a department head and supervisor and as an activity leader. This is not to suggest that activity coordinators should not continue to work directly with residents. They should, but the amount of time spent directly with residents and the kinds of things done with residents needs to change.

In the relatively short history of comprehensive activity programs in long term care facilities, which only dates back to the late 1960s with the implementation of the initial Medicare regulations, activity programs have grown tremendously. According to Maypole,

As a profession into which its members have come with a wide variety of skill levels and educational backgrounds, activity [coordination] has been slowly gaining more recognition and acceptance. This acceptance is primarily reflected in the federal and state laws and regulations which require (1) organized activity . . . programs in nursing homes and (2) the participation of the activity (professional) in the care plan conferences and programming. However, having no common theoretical or educational base for its members, the profession is only now beginning to grapple with developing job performance standards and uniform educational expectations. (1985, p. 15)

The concept of an activity program as originally understood by administrators, nurses, and even surveyors was one in which activities staff provided entertainment-oriented activities to keep the residents busy and happy. The common view was that activities were something that were nice, but not very important to the quality of the long term care facility. An activity department was simply one more requirement which needed to be met in order to receive reimbursement through Medicare and Medicaid.

During the twenty some years since those beginnings, activity programs have become a mandated part of the resident's care plan, and the nature and variety of the activities which are a part of the program have changed and grown dramatically. Activities are offered not merely as entertainment, but for specific treatment purposes. The activity program requirements are now a more substantive part of federal and state regulations to the place where facilities are now cited for deficiencies in their activity programs. For example, regulations in Oregon state,

An activity program shall be provided which is suited to the intellectual, social, spiritual, creative, and physical need(s), capabilities, and interests of the patients which encourages involvement and allows the patients to function at their highest level. This program shall be provided as an important part of the treatment program and coordinated with the overall plan of care. . . . There shall be an activity plan developed for each patient based on the total patient assessment including, but not limited to, past and current interests and activities, skills, medical limitations, cognitive and emotional functioning . . . The goal(s) and plan shall be entered on the overall plan of care. (Oregon Health Division, 1985)

While it is not pleasant to receive citations for deficiencies in activities, they represent dramatic acknowledgement of the greater importance of activity programs, especially from the perspective of surveyors.

The amount of growth and development in what is a very short professional history is truly phenomenal. Much of the credit goes to the hard work of current and former activity professionals. But the acceptance of activity programs by administrators and other staff has not changed as much as the developments discussed above might have warranted. As Dickey (1986) has stated, "I have had numerous activity directors tell me that they are at the bottom as far as the administrative staff is considered. I have heard this from people with schooling, with experience" (p. 79).

Two reasons for the lack of acceptance seem most likely. The first may be reflective of the nature of activity programs and the professional competence of activity coordinators. Leisure activities are, first of all, fun for the participants, and many do not feel that fun is very important to the quality of living of people. While activities certainly do provide pleasure and enjoyment for participants, their purposes in meeting physical, intellectual, emotional, social, and spiritual needs are much deeper than they appear. However, documenting the effects of the activity program on residents through research is also a critical need, and activity coordinators must begin to initiate and/or work with researchers to collect information which specifically addresses the efficacy of the activity program.

Additionally, planning, organizing, and implementing pleasurable experiences do not, on the surface, appear to be very hard work. How many times have activity coordinators heard other staff members say "I wish I had your job. All you do is play all day?" Those who plan and implement activities all know the amount of time, energy, and skills that are required, but perhaps because activity coordinators do their jobs so well and so professionally, the work does not appear to be that difficult or demanding.

A second, and more important, reason for lack of acceptance appears to be that activity coordinators frequently don't view and conduct themselves as department heads and supervisors. Dickey continues, "I think that how we feel about ourselves and our departments is vital in establishing professionalism" (1986, p. 79). Too often, activity coordinators are not assertive in promoting the activity program to the administrator and other staff. Too often, when lack of support from the administrator and other staff occurs, activity coordinators do not confront them. Instead, they go along doing their jobs and hope others will somehow notice how important the activity program is to the residents.

Maypole's (1985) study of activity professionals' perceptions of their continuing education needs suggests that they do not view themselves as department heads and supervisors. The majority of higher priority training needs included many topics related specifically to working directly with residents (e.g., working with confused residents, bedfast activities, motivating individuals, working with groups, special mental health problems, helping techniques with death and dying, and leadership techniques). More of the perceived lower priority training needs were related to administration (e.g., volunteer recruitment, volunteer use, newspaper releases, TV publicity, appraising supervisees, delegating, budgeting, planning, evaluating job applications) even when practice and administrative needs were separated.

When the activity coordinator begins to view her or himself as a department head and supervisor and functions accordingly, greater acceptance and recognition will come. Even through assuming this new role as a department head may not initially be very comfortable, the basic reason for doing so is to provide the residents with the type of activity program which gives their lives greater meaning and helps them to feel good about themselves and what they can do for themselves and others. Enhancing the quality of living of the residents surely is justification enough for any activity coordinator beginning to view her or himself and function as a department head and supervisor.

DETERMINING
THE MOST EFFECTIVE
SUPERVISORY STYLE

Once the activity coordinator has begun to view her or himself as a department head and supervisor, it is, of course, essential that she or he learns how to become an effective supervisor. Essentially, effective supervision represents effective leadership of subordinate staff.

A variety of research has been conducted in an effort to determine the characteristics of the effective leader or supervisor. Edginton and Williams (1978, p. 180) conclude, "In most cases, leadership behavior studies have found that the critical elements are task behavior and relationship [people-oriented] behavior." Kraus (1985) supports this conclusion and goes on to describe *task-oriented* (supervisors) as primarily concerned with the work to be done who receive their chief satisfaction from work accomplishment and *person-oriented* [supervisors] as those who emphasize interpersonal relationships more than they do task accomplishment (p. 44).

"The most desirable leadership style has equal concern for people and product [task]" (Edginton and Williams, 1978, pp. 181-182). According to Blake and Mouton (1978), supervisors who rank high in both a concern for people and a concern for the tasks to be accomplished develop employees who have a sense of interdependence and commitment to accomplishing the goals of the organization through their work in an atmosphere of trust and respect. Ideally, then, the most effective supervision by an activity coordinator focuses equally on the tasks which must be completed by activity assistants and others and the morale of these employees and volunteers. The ultimate goal is to supervise in such a way that both high productivity and high morale result.

Applying this ideal to selecting the most effective supervisory style for an individual activity coordinator, in a specific facility, and in relationship to specific issues, however, requires an examination of three factors.

1. *The supervisor*: the individual supervisor's personality, including her or his value system and supervisory inclinations;
2. *The subordinate(s)*: the individual subordinate's personality, including individual values, need for independence, readiness to assume responsibility, tolerance for ambiguity, degree of commitment to the goals of the facility, expectations of shared decision-making, and experience and expertise, and the combined effects of these issues if there is more than one activity assistant; and
3. *Organizational environment*: the characteristics of the facility, including size of the facility and the activity department, type of issue being addressed, pressure of time to make decisions, and amount and type of authority of the activity coordinator (Tannenbaum and Schmidt, 1958, pp. 98-101).

The most effective supervisory style, then, will be dependent on an analysis of these three factors. The activity coordinator will need to remain flexible and able to adapt to a given situation if she or he is to be an effective supervisor since no one style will be effective in all situations.

THE ELEMENTS
OF EMPLOYING AND SUPERVISING
ACTIVITY ASSISTANTS AND OTHERS

A number of elements are essential to hiring, supervising, and evaluating activity assistants and working with other staff. Each of these elements needs to be thoroughly addressed if supervision is to be successful.

Hiring the Right Person
to Be an Activity Assistant

Learning how to hire and orient activity assistants is a challenging task. Careful attention to a number of elements will make success more likely. These include: developing a thorough job description, being aware of sources for recruiting activity assistants, knowing how to select the best applicant, and orienting the new activity assistant in such a way that she or he is ready and able to meet the requirements of the position.

Job Description. Figure 1 is an example of a job description for an activity assistant. This job description is presented as an example and is not the definitive description for all activity assistant positions. It is important that a job description be developed which reflects the specific facility and activity program for which an activity assistant is being employed.

Any job description should include the job title, a concise statement of the overall purpose of the job, a listing of specific duties; and a statement of by whom the employee is supervised and who the employee supervises (Armstrong, 1988, pp. 167-168). For activity assistant positions, it is also helpful to include required knowledge, skills, and abilities. In order to recruit and employ the best activity assistant possible, it is essential that the responsibilities of the position are thoroughly delineated and understood by all parties involved in the process. Since the responsibilities of an activity assistant are many and varied, it is always wise to include "other duties as assigned by the activity coordinator" as one of the specific duties. A thorough and available job description will be of assistance in eliminating problems with activity assistants after they have been employed.

Sources of Activity Assistants. Although an ad should be placed in the local newspaper(s) in order to recruit an activity assistant, a variety of other potential sources should be explored. These include: near-by community colleges and universities, local activity coordinator organizations, and local human service agencies and organizations. Although these sources should be tapped, perhaps the best way to locate potential activity assistants is through word of mouth. The activity coordinator should talk with volunteers and others in the community to inform them of the available position.

Selecting the Best Applicant

Selecting is, at best, a difficult process because it involves making judgements about people. Three essential questions must be answered if the most qualified person is to be selected. These questions are: What is the applicant's "can do"

Figure 1. Sample Job Description for an Activity Assistant

JOB DESCRIPTION: Activity Assistant

Overall Responsibilities: To assist the Activity Coordinator in the organization, development, and maintenance of the facility activity program.

Specific Duties:
1. Organize and implement specific activities as assigned by the Activity Coordinator
2. Implement community outings following policies and procedures for van use
3. Start activities on time in accordance with activity calendars
4. Prepare and mount monthly activity calendars and distribute weekly calendars according to established deadlines and procedures
5. Maintain accurate daily attendance records of individual resident participation in activities
6. Remind residents and staff early of activity programs through invitation and the PA system
7. Assist with transporting residents to and from activities
8. Arrange rooms and collect necessary equipment and supplies for activity programs
9. Secure substitutions for program cancellations
10. Contribute to resident care plans through memos or conferences with the Activity Coordinator
11. Direct and assist volunteers as assigned by the Activity Coordinator
12. Monitor inventory of equipment and supplies, informing Activity Coordinator of needs
13. Maintain equipment and supplies
14. Purchase supplies with the approval of the Activity Coordinaotr
15. Attend in-service training sessions and the 36-hour basic course when available
16. Participate in department meetings with the Activity Coordinator
17. Complete reading assigned by the Activity Coordinator
18. Complete other tasks as assigned by the Activity Coordinator

Required Knowledge, Skills, and Abilities:

--creative

--reliable

--flexible

--ability to work effectively with people

--ability to plan and organize leisure activities

--desire to work with older people and people with disabilities

--understanding of the needs of older people and people with disabilities

--patient

--tactful

--enthusiastic

--ability to deal with residents at whatever cognitive or physical level they may be

--willingness to learn

--ability to work under supervision and independently

--self starter

--willingness to work a flexible and occasionally extended schedule

--ability to delegate to and supervise volunteers

Supervision: The Activity Assistant is responsible to the Activity Coordinator
The Activity Assistant supervises volunteers

I have read the above job description, fully understand the duties of the position, and will perform these duties to the best of my ability.

Signed: _____

Activity Assistant   Date

_____

Activity Coordinator   Date

ability? What is the applicant's "will do" ability? How will the applicant "fit" into the organization? "Can do" ability refers to experience and education required to perform a specific job; "will do" ability refers to the level of motivation the person will actually exert in performing the job; "fit" refers to how well the individual will conform to the socio-psychological environment of the organization. (Caruth, Noe, and Mondy, 1988, p. 149)

The application materials (resume, completed application form, and references) of all applicants should be reviewed to select those who will be interviewed. Applicants who do not meet the qualifications for the position should be eliminated since interviewing is a time-consuming process.

A thorough interview is essential to selecting the most qualified applicant for an activity assistant position. In many cases, interviews do not predict job performance because they are not well-planned. "Research has shown that interviews that follow a semi-structured format and employ an interview guide, a list of all relevant questions to be asked of each candidate, tend to have a reasonable degree of validity and reliability" (Culkin and Kirsch, 1986, p. 121). Culkin and Kirsch recommend the following interview steps for each applicant:

1. Begin the interview with a brief period of small talk;
2. Tell the applicant what the format of the interview will be;
3. Provide the applicant with information about the job, including duties, salary, benefits, and any undesirable aspects of the job [for example, sometimes working evenings and weekends];
4. Follow the interview guide of questions to gather information from the interviewee;
5. Allow the applicant a chance to ask questions; and
6. Close the interview, explaining what happens next in the selection process, when a decision will be made, and when the applicant will hear from you (1986, p. 123).

Applicants should be interviewed primarily by the activity coordinator, but an interview by the administrator to obtain additional perspective is also helpful.

Additionally, a great deal of information about an applicant can be learned informally during conversations as the facility is toured and activities observed. It is important to pay particular attention to the applicant's reactions to residents, especially those who are low functioning. Does the applicant appear comfortable? Does the applicant interact with residents when, inevitably during a tour, some will talk with the activity coordinator and perhaps inquire about the applicant?

A great deal more can be learned about each applicant if she or he is asked to assist with an activity as a regular part of the interview process. In this way, actual skills, abilities, and reactions can be carefully observed.

All of the information available about each applicant interviewed should then be reviewed including the information provided on resumes and application forms, gathered from references, collected during interviews, and obtained informally while applicants were at the facility for interviews. It is especially important that references provided by each applicant be contacted, as well as any previous supervisor who may not have been listed as a reference.

While the ultimate selection decision should be made by the activity coordinator, it is wise to seek the opinions of other staff who interviewed or interacted with the applicants. Selection should be based primarily on an objective evaluation of the information gathered on each applicant, but it is also important to include intuitive or "gut level" reactions to applicants since the activity coordinator and the activity assistant must work closely together, frequently in highly stressful situations, in order to plan and operate the activity program.

Unfortunately, because of low salaries and a lack of understanding of what an activity assistant does, the activity coordinator does not always have many qualified applicants from which to select an activity assistant. Occasionally, it is necessary to select the best person available, who may not be well-qualified, for the position. In this situation, a more careful orientation, more thorough on-going training, and closer supervision of the activity assistant may well be necessary.

Orientation of Activity Assistants and Other Staff

Thoroughly orienting activity assistants and other staff will contribute significantly to greater competence and understanding. "An effective orientation program can significantly increase employee satisfaction and reduce turnover" (Holley and Jennings as reported in Culkin and Kirsch, 1986, p. 126).

Orientation of Activity Assistants. A thorough orientation is essential if the activity assistant is to be enabled to complete job responsibilities effectively. An Orientation and Training Checklist for activity assistants is presented in Figure 2.

The Checklist includes: a space to indicate that the job description has been signed; sections delineating information to be covered in the categories of administration, programs, and documentation; and spaces for the signatures of both the activity assistant and the activity coordinator indicating that the listed information has been covered in the orientation.

Orientation of Other Employees to the Activity Program. It is imperative that all new staff, but especially nursing staff, be oriented to the activity program for at least two reasons. First, the activity program and the responsibilities of activities staff are frequently misunderstood by other staff. As was discussed earlier, the purposes of the activity program and the time and effort necessary to plan and conduct the program are not always apparent. Second, it is not possible to conduct an effective activity program without the support and assistance of other staff. Time spent thoroughly orienting and establishing rapport with new staff in all disciplines is time well spent which will, in the long run, pay large dividends to the activity program.

The orientation of other staff should include written information for each individual and sessions with the activity coordinator. Written and oral information should focus on two general areas, both of which should be covered in some detail.

1. The *purposes and role of the activity program* including its therapeutic aspects, from both an overall and individual resident perspective

   — contributes significantly to quality of living of the resident
   — activities determined by the needs and interests of the resident
   — provision to meet physical, emotional, intellectual, social, creative, and spiritual needs of the resident
   — provision for empowerment of the resident including opportunities for choices
   — availability of and the use of activity calendars
   — bedside activities
   — the importance and role of volunteers including positive interaction with and appreciation of them
   — the use of individual care plans to obtain information about activity plans

2. The *importance of teamwork* to the success of the activity program and the quality of living of residents

   — encouragement of residents to participate in activities
   — participation by staff in activities
   — communication of the needs and responses of residents
   — transportation of residents to and from activities

On-Going Supervision and Training of the Activity Assistant

Once an activity assistant has been employed and oriented, the activity coordinator will need to provide the kind of on-going supervision which results in both high productivity and high morale. The key to effective supervision is to find ways to motivate the activity assistant. Ideally, supervision will be such that the activity assistant becomes self-motivated, so that constant direction is not required. According to Edginton and Williams (1978, pp. 84-85), motivation is a function of four factors: *needs, opportunity, ability,* and *reinforcement.*

Figure 2. Sample Orientation and Training Checklist for an Activity Assistant

<u>ACTIVITY ASSISTANT ORIENTATION AND TRAINING CHECKLIST</u>

____ JOB DESCRIPTION SIGNED

ADMINISTRATION OF THE ACTIVITY DEPARTMENT

____ 1. Review Policies and Procedures Manual, including the importance of state and federal regulations

____ 2. Scheduling weekly meetings with the Activity Coordinator

____ 3. Maintenance of resident participation attendance records

____ 4. Care of equipment and supplies

____ 5. Disinfection of equipment as scheduled

____ 6. Use of time clock and sign-in procedures

____ 7. Participation in continuing education

____ 9. Review of fire drill, disaster plan, and other safety regulations

____ 10. Use of and policies and procedures for use of the facility van

____ 11. Assistance with transporting residents to and from activities

____ 12. Preparation and maintenance of activity areas

____ 13. Procedures for special events

____ 14. Operating programs as scheduled; obtaining substitutions for cancellations

____ 15. Preparation and distribution of monthly and weekly activities calendars

____ 16. Procedures for working with and directing volunteers

____ 17. Assistance and follow-up with resident volunteers

____ 18. Instruction of volunteers on special diets

____ 19. Maintaining the image of the Activity Department in the facility and the community

___ 20. Relationships with other staff (administrator, department heads, nursing assistants, dietary, maintenance, and others)

___ 21. Procedures for arranging activities requiring communication with other departments

ACTIVITY PROGRAMS

___ 1. Therapeutic programming
___ 2. Activities with physical goals
___ 3. Activities for cognitive stimulation
___ 4. Activities with spiritual goals
___ 5. Activities with cultural goals
___ 6. Activities with social/interaction goals
___ 7. Activities for the lower functioning resident
___ 8. Activities for the socially/self isolated resident
___ 9. Bedside and one-to-one activities
___ 10. Special events

DOCUMENTATION

___ 1. Orientation to care plans
___ 2. Census update (new admits and discharges)
___ 3. Contributing to care planning
___ 4. Instruction in documentation

Signed: _____ _____ _____ _____
         Activity Assistant   Date   Activity Coordinator   Date

First, motivation is a function of meeting the *needs* of employees. Herzberg, Mausner, and Snyderman (1959) conducted a classic study which examined motivation of workers which continues to be widely quoted in the management literature. They concluded that employees have two categories of needs that are met through their work. *Hygiene factors* include needs which are not an integral part of the job (e.g., salary, fringe benefits, working conditions, job security, type of supervision, and interpersonal relationships with others [supervisors, co-workers, and subordinates]). If hygiene factors are not provided for, workers will be dissatisfied with their jobs, and their work will be affected. Hygiene factors can be especially important with activity assistants since low salaries and other factors can sometimes result in poor performance and resignations. However, hygiene factors do not, in themselves, motivate workers or result in satisfaction with a job. The second category of needs is termed *motivators* by Herzberg. These motivators (e.g., achievement, recognition for one's accomplishments, responsibility, advancement, possibility of growth, and challenging work), when they are provided, create job satisfaction in workers and often result in increased work output. Hygiene factors, then, are important as a basis for motivating workers, but they do not motivate them. Given that hygiene factors are present in the job of the activity assistant, the activity coordinator must focus on the motivators listed above to increase productivity and morale.

Second, motivation is a function of *opportunity*. To motivate activity assistants, the activity coordinator must create opportunities for them. These include opportunities such as providing greater freedom and greater variety as a part of the job, increasing involvement in decision-making, and providing chances to participate in continuing education experiences. Opportunity may also mean that the activity assistant moves to an activity coordinator position at another facility when that becomes available which was discussed earlier. Activity assistants should have a variety of opportunities as they become more proficient in the position if they are to continue to be motivated.

The third function of motivation is *ability*. This includes providing supervision and training so that the activity assistant is able to meet the responsibilities of the position. The activity coordinator should meet weekly with the activity assistant to provide training for the position on an on-going basis. Although the training needs of individual activity assistants will vary, topics covered might include: working with older people, working with low functioning and socially isolated residents, common health conditions of residents, dealing with resident behavior problems, orientation to specific activities, working with other staff, working with volunteers, how to efficiently provide the information needed for documentation, and new information as it becomes available. In addition to individual training provided by the activity coordinator to enhance the ability of the activity assistant, other continuing education opportunities should be provided which include taking the basic 36-hour course when it is available and participation in other external workshops and conferences and facility in-service training sessions.

Reinforcement is the fourth function of motivation. It is almost always best to provide positive (e.g., praise and recognition for doing a job well, greater job security, salary increases, opportunities for advancement, employee development opportunities, involvement in decision-making, greater freedom in work) rather than negative reinforcement (e.g., criticism, close supervision, reprimands). Positive reinforcement is generally more effective with employees. Negative reinforcement should only be used when positive reinforcement has not been effective although employees do need to understand through constructive criticism the things they may not be doing correctly.

Each of the four functions of motivation discussed above may involve the *delegation of responsibilities to the activity assistant*. Since the activity coordinator has typically been the only employee primarily responsible for activities, delegation may be especially difficult. More generally, delegation by most supervisors is frequently not effective (Bannon, 1981, p. 10).

There are a number of reasons why this is the case. Managers may be reluctant to delegate authority because they do not have confidence in their employees or they are unwilling to take the "risk" that this may involve. They may fail to understand the advantages of successful delegation, or may have a desire for nothing "short of perfection." On the other hand, they may fear to delegate because they are unwilling to give up the reins of power or because they fear that employees will "outshine" them by doing the tasks too well. (Kraus, 1985, p. 48)

Stewart (1986) suggests two benefits to the supervisor which result from good delegating skills. First, delegating routine tasks gives supervisors the time to perform management functions. A second benefit is that delegation can contribute to employee development and job enrichment (pp. 77-78). Considering the need for activity coordinators to begin to function as department heads, developing and implementing delegation skills is essential to assuming this new role.

Working Effectively with Other Staff

The information presented above concerning the supervision and motivation of activity assistants applies, for the most part, to finding ways to work effectively with other staff, especially nursing staff. Other staff can also become motivated to work more cooperatively with activity program staff through the implementation of four factors discussed. The activity coordinator can work to meet the *needs* of other staff by addressing motivators, such as recognition for cooperation and assistance. The activity coordinator can work with supervisors to provide especially helpful staff with *opportunities* to participate in activities, especially community outings, and *ability* through continuing education experiences. Lastly, the activity coordinator can provide positive *reinforcement* to other staff for cooperation and assistance through such things as praise and recognition through awards.

Performance Appraisal of Activity Assistants

As is true for all employees, activity assistants should receive periodic performance appraisals. Performance appraisals serve several important functions:

1. Provide input into administrative decisions such a raises and retention;
2. Motivate employees to higher performance and goal-setting;
3. Identify training needs by locating employee deficiencies as early as possible; and
4. Provides legal documentation of performance problems of marginal employees (Stewart, 1986, pp. 229-230).

Although specific criteria for evaluating activity assistants should be developed to reflect individual positions, the following criteria, based upon the experiences of the authors, provide suggestions on which to base performance appraisals:

1. Knowledge of the job

   – Understands the duties, responsibilities, and procedures involved in the work

2. Dependability

   – Programs are provided in accordance with established procedures and as scheduled
   – Is punctual and dependable in attendance

3. Productivity

   – Amount of work produced compares favorably with the expectations of the assignment

4. Quality of work

   – Values accuracy
   – Values thoroughness and neatness
   – Handles unexpected situations and changing circumstances professionally
   – Reacts calmly to emergency situations
   – Works well with limited supervision
   – Recommends alternative ways of doing things
   – Maintains equipment
   – Observes all safety rules

5. Relationships with staff, residents, and families

   – Uses tact

— Is patient and understanding
— Responds effectively and professionally

6. Initiative

— Willing to learn new responsibilities
— Provides assistance when need is apparent
— Seeks additional knowledge and information
— Is a self-starter
— Asks questions when in doubt

7. Attitude toward supervision and direction

— Accepts supervision and direction willingly
— Follows directions effectively

The performance appraisal form should also include a narrative summary of the major strengths of the activity assistant and a narrative summary of the areas in need of improvement for both the short and long terms. In addition, the activity assistant should have space to provide any comments on the completed evaluation. Spaces for the signatures of the activity assistant, activity coordinator, and the administrator, as well as the date, should also be provided.

Performance appraisal should ideally be a two-way process. An especially effective method is to have both the supervisor and the employee independently evaluate the job performance of the employee and then meet to compare evaluations and, hopefully, find agreement.

Occasionally, the job performance of activity assistants does not meet minimum standards for the position. Culkin and Kirsch (1986) recommend a careful sequence of steps which should be taken in an effort to improve job performance before termination is considered. In a situation in which employees belong to a union, it is essential that all contracts and agreements be carefully examined in order to specifically follow established procedures for substandard performance.

1. *Counseling techniques* should be used by the supervisor in an effort to determine the reasons for substandard performance or misconduct.
2. An *oral warning* through which the employee is told that sub-

standard performance must be improved or the misconduct corrected and what the penalty will be if the behavior is not corrected is the next step if counseling techniques are not effective.

3. A *reprimand* or written warning is a formal record of a disciplinary interview with the employee. The written warning should contain all the major areas discussed during the interview, expected improvement in behavior, and the nature of the reprimand. Everyone present signs the dated form, one copy is given to the employee, and another copy is placed in the employee's personnel file.

4. *Suspension* or leave without pay may be used as the next step, but this is not often used with while-collar employees.

5. *Discharge* may be the final step if the employee's performance has not improved or the employee has not resigned (pp. 252-255).

Most often, disciplinary action will not be necessary, however, if open and honest efforts are made to resolve problems and issues as early as possible. Stewart (1986) recommends a four step process in dealing with conflict more generally, including problems with employees.

1. *Clearly identify the conflict or problem.* The supervisor may need to search below the surface to determine the true cause of the conflict or problem.

2. *Openly communicate.* The supervisor must make certain that communication is open among all parties involved, and that the conflict or problem is clearly understood by all parties involved.

3. *Negotiate a solution.* The supervisor should negotiate a resolution that is the best solution possible for all parties involved under the given circumstances. The negotiated solution must be seen as fair by all parties.

4. *Implement the negotiated solution.* While this step may seem obvious, it is often more difficult than negotiating a solution. It is at this step that changes must actually be made if the problem or conflict is to be resolved. If the solution is not

implemented, the negotiation may be seen as having been in bad faith which will create additional problems and conflicts (pp. 142-144).

It is important to recognize that conflict is inevitable in any organization or program if that organization or program is growing and developing. As Stewart states,

Lack of conflict in an organization may also indicate that no new ideas are being tried, no new approaches investigated, no one daring to make waves. Such a static organization may fall victim to the first major change that comes along. The price of creativity and innovation is often conflict. (1986, p. 142)

CONCLUSIONS

Activity programs in long term care facilities have grown tremendously during their relatively short history since the late 1960s. They are more specifically delineated in the regulations, an integral part of the care plans of residents, have specific treatment-oriented purposes, and include a wider variety of activities. However, acceptance of activities by administrators and other staff, as having an integral role in the quality of the lives of residents and the quality of the overall facility, lags behind these advances. The major reason for this situation may be that activity coordinators have not viewed themselves or functioned primarily as department heads and supervisors rather than activity leaders.

Activity coordinators need to extend their considerable abilities and skills as far as possible. The most effective way to extend those abilities is to supervise activity assistants, volunteers, and other staff as they become the primary direct leaders of activity programs.

Learning to be an effective supervisor begins with the activity coordinator viewing her or himself as a department head. Once this self-concept is established, the activity coordinator can learn to be an effective supervisor through examining different supervisory styles and adopting the one that is likely to be most effective in a given situation. Supervisory effectiveness can be further developed through using specific procedures to employ the best activity assistants and supervise them and other staff in such a way that they become self-motivated. This can best be accomplished through meeting the needs of staff supervised, enhancing their abilities through training and continuing education, providing opportunities for professional development, and reinforcing efforts positively whenever possible.

There are two reasons why it is essential for an activity coordinator to function primarily as a department head and supervisor. First, the facility will have the kind of activity program which creates a positive image in the community, and second and more importantly, which contributes significantly to residents having the highest quality of living possible.

REFERENCES

Armstrong, M. (1988). *A handbook of personnel management practice*. New York: Nichols Press.

Bannon, J.J. (1981). *Problem-solving in recreation and parks*. Englewood Cliffs, NJ: Prentice-Hall.

Blake, R., & Mouton, J.S. (1978). *The new management grid*. Houston, TX: Gulf Publishing.

Caruth, D.L., Noe, R.M., & Mondy, R.W. (1988). *Staffing the contemporary organization*. New York: Quorum Books.

Culkin, D.F., & Kirsch, S.L. (1986). *Managing human resources in recreation, parks, and leisure services*. New York: Macmillan.

Dickey, H. (1986). What is an activity professional? *Activities, Adaptation & Aging, 9* (1), 79-83.

Edginton, C.R., & Williams, J.G. (1978). *Productive management of leisure service organizations*. New York: John Wiley.

Herzberg, F., Mausner, B., & Snyderman, B. (1959). *The motivation to work*. New York: John Wiley.

Kraus, R.G. (1985). *Recreation leadership today*. Glenview, IL: Scott-Foresman.

Maypole, D.E. (1985). Activity therapist continuing education needs assessment. *Activities, Adaptation & Aging, 7* (2), 15-23.

Oregon Health Division. (1985, November). Patient activities regulations. Chapter 333, Division 867.

Stewart, D. (1986). *The power of people skills*. New York: John Wiley.

Tannenbaum, R., & Schmidt, W.G. (1958). How to chose a leadership pattern. *Harvard Business review, 36* (2), 95-102.

AGING AND LEISURE BIBLIOGRAPHY

The Aging and Leisure Bibliography is published twice a year in *Activities, Adaptation & Aging*. It is intended to serve researchers, leisure service personnel, activity directors, and others working with older adults. Over fifty journals and publications are reviewed in compiling this bibliography. Entries are divided into fifteen categories and are not generally cross-referenced. The reader is advised to review all appropriate categories. Breadth of resources reviewed and timeliness are major goals of the bibliography.

Ted Tedrick, Editor
Temple University

The following individuals are contributors to the Aging and Leisure Bibliography: Michael Blazey, Washington State University; Patricia Johnson Brown, Virginia Commonwealth University; Mary D'Urso, Temple University; Regina B. Glover, Southern Illinois University; M. Jean Keller, North Texas State University; Richard MacNeil, University of Iowa; Francis McGuire, Clemson University; B.J. McNeillie, Temple University; Ken Mobily, University of Iowa; Sandy Parker, Western Illinois University; George Patrick, National Institute of Health; Jerome Singleton, Dalhousie University; Richard Smith, Miami (Ohio) University; Michael Teague, University of Iowa; Ted Tedrick, Temple University; Carlton S. VanDoren, Texas A & M University.

Thanks is extended to Carol Gallup, Temple University, for typing the Bibliography.

SECTION I
PROGRAMMING, INNOVATIVE PROGRAMS,
EFFECTS OF LEISURE PROGRAMS, THERAPIES

Alessio, H.M., Grier, L.J., & Leviton, D. (1989). Trailblazing recreational programming for the elderly: High-risk activities. *Activities, Adaptation & Aging, 13*(4), 9-16.

Bentel, M.J. (1989). Who are you supposed to be? *Activities, Adaptation & Aging, 13*(4), 31-32.

Buettner, L. (1988). Utilizing development theory and adaptive equipment with regressed geriatric patients in therapeutic recreation. *Therapeutic Recreation Journal,* 22(3), 72-79.

Dottavio, F.D., McGuire, F.A. & O'Leary, J.T. (1989). The importance of selected facilities, programs, and services to older visitors to national parks. *Journal of Park and Recreation Administration, 17*(3), 1-9.

Forsythe, E. (1988/89). One-to-one therapeutic recreation activities for the bed and/or room bound. *Activities, Adaptation & Aging, 13*(1/2), 63-76.

Gillespie, K.A., Kennedy, D.W., & Soble, K. (1988/89). Utilizing importance-performance analysis in the evaluation and marketing of activity programs in geriatric settings. *Activities, Adaptation & Aging, 13*(1/2), 77-89.

Hillebrand, W.U. (1988/89). Residents' newsletter as a therapeutic tool. *Activities, Adaptation & Aging, 13*(1/2), 51-61.

Mahalski, P., Jones, R., and Maxwell, G. (1988). The value of cat ownership to elderly women living alone. *International Journal of Aging and Human Development,* 27(4), 249-260.

McMurray, J. (1989). Creative arts with older people. *Activities, Adaptation & Aging, 14*(1/2), 1-138.

Peck, C.F. (1989). From deep within: Poetry workshops in nursing homes. *Activities, Adaptation & Aging, 13*(3), 1-153.

Robertson, R. (1988). Recreation and the institutionalized elderly: Conceptualization of the free choice and intervention continuum. *Activities, Adaptation & Aging, 11*(1), 61-73.

Shour, A. (1988/89). A residents' newsletter: Social action and power. *Activities, Adaptation & Aging, 13*(1/2), 43-49.

White, S. and Landis, L. (1989, November-December). Designing aquatic exercise programs – Three guiding principles, *Journal of Physical Education, Recreation, and Dance*, *60*(9), 40-42.

Williams, J. (1988/89). Enabling the Alzheimer's "Person." *Activities, Adaptation & Aging*, *13*(1/2), 25-28.

SECTION II
LIFE SATISFACTION, QUALITY OF LIFE, WELL BEING, LEISURE AS A VARIABLE IN LIFE SATISFACTION

Adams, R. (1988). Which comes first: Poor psychological well-being or decreased friendship activity? *Activities, Adaptation & Aging*, *12*(1-2), 27-41.

Beck, S. and Page, J. (1988). Involvement in activities and the psychological well-being of retired men. *Activities, Adaptation & Aging*, *11*(1), 31-47.

Bishop, D., Epstein, N., Baldwin, L., Miller, I. and Keitner, G. (1988). Older couples: The effect of health, retirement, and family functioning on morale. *Family Systems Medicine*, *6*(2), 238-247.

Brown, W. and Brown, D. (1988). Enhancing life satisfaction for older adults. *Journal of Applied Sociology*, *5*, 73-87.

Card, J.A. (1988/89). Perceived leisure functioning of nursing home patients: Does recreation make a difference? *Activities, Adaptation & Aging*, *13*(1/2), 29-40.

Clark, P. (1988). Autonomy, personal empowerment, and quality of life in long-term care. *Journal of Applied Gerontology*, *7*(3), 279-297.

Faulk, L. (1988). Quality of life factors in board and care homes for the elderly: A hierarchical model. *Adult Foster Care Journal*, *2*(2), 100-117.

Ishii-Kuntz, M. (1990). Social interaction and psychological well-being: Comparison across stages of adulthood. *International Journal of Aging and Human Development*. *30*(1), 15-36.

Kelly, J.R. and Ross, J. (1989). Later-life leisure: Beginning a new agenda. *Leisure Sciences*, *11*(1), 47-59.

Maynard, M. (1988/89). Health maintenance through stress management: A wellness approach for elderly clients. *Activities, Adaptation & Aging, 13*(1/2), 117-127.

McConatha, J.T. & McConatha, P.D. (1988/89). The study of the relationship between wellness and life satisfaction of older adults. *Activities, Adaptation & Aging, 13*(1/2), 129-140.

Purcell, R.Z. & Keller, M.J. (1989). Characteristics of leisure activities which may lead to leisure satisfaction among older adults. *Activities, Adaptation & Aging, 13*(4), 17-29.

Tokarski, W. (1989, Spring). Continuity and discontinuity of leisure lifestyles in old age: Results of a reanalysis. *World Leisure and Recreation, 31*(1), 27-28.

SECTION III
TIME USE, PARTICIPATION PATTERNS, TRAVEL AND TOURISM, RESEARCH ISSUES

Goodfellow, M., Kierman, N.E., Ahern, F. and Smoyer, M. (1988). Response bias using two-stage data collection: A study of elderly participants in a program. *Evaluation Review, 12*(6), 638-654.

Hawes, D. (1988). Travel-related lifestyle profiles of older women. *Journal of Travel Research. 27*, (2).

Shoemaker, S. (1989). Segmentation of the senior pleasure travel market. *Journal of Travel Research.* (27)3.

Teaff, J. and Hamilton, K. (1988). The psychological benefits of elderly recreational travel. *Leisure Information Quarterly, 14*(3), 8-10.

Voelkl, J. and Birkel, R. (1988). Application of the experience sampling method to assess clients' daily experiences. *Therapeutic Recreation Journal, 22*(3), 23-33.

Wingrove, C.R. (1987). Some considerations in interviewing the old, old. *Mid-American Review of Sociology, 12*(2), 71-76.

SECTION IV
RETIREMENT, LEISURE AS A PART OF RETIREMENT, WORK, RETIREMENT COMMUNITIES, PLANNING FOR RETIREMENT

DeViney, S. and O'Rand, A. (1988). Gender-cohort succession and retirement among older men and women, 1951-1984. *The Sociological Quarterly, 29*(4), 525-540.

Ferraro, K. (1989). The ADEA amendment and public support for older workers. *Research on Aging, 11*(1), 53-81.

Hayward, M., Grady, W. and McLaughlin, S. (1988). The retirement process among older women in the United States. *Research on Aging*, 10(3), 358-382.

Hogarth, J.M. (1989). Models of accepting an early retirement incentive. *Lifestyles – Family and Economic Issues, 10*(1), 61-82.

Hunnicut, B. (1988). Work, leisure, and labor supply: An analysis of the 1980 U.S. Census Data. *International Review of Modern Sociology, 18*(1), 31-55.

Kaye, L. and Monk, A. (1989). College educators and the retirement decision. *Educational Gerontology, 15*(5), 543-555.

Khullar, G.S. (1989). Retirement and organizational participation of older males. *Activities, Adaptation & Aging, 13*(4), 55-70.

Khullar, G. (1988). Retirement social participation and social integration. *International Review of Modern Sociology, 18*(2), 107-137.

Morris, R. and Bass, S. (1988). A new class in America: A revisionist view of retirement. *Social Policy, 18*(4), 38-43.

Morrow-Howell, N. and Leon, J. (1988). Life-span determinants of work in retirement years. *International Journal of Aging and Human Development, 27*(2), 125-140.

Searle, M. and Iso-Ahola, S. (1988). Determinants of leisure behavior among retired adults. *Therapeutic Recreation Journal, 22*(2), 38-46.

Voges, W. and Pongratz, H. (1988). Retirement and the lifestyles of older women. *Aging and Society, 8*(1), 63-83.

SECTION V
LIVING ENVIRONMENT,
ACTIVITY AND LEISURE ENVIRONMENT

Meyer, J.W. and Cromley, E.K. (1989, November). Caregiving environments and elderly residential mobility. *The Professional Geographer, 41*(4), 440-450.
Wister, A.V. (1989). Environmental adaptation by persons in their later life. *Research on Aging, 11*(3), 267-291.

SECTION VI
ROLE OF FAMILY, SUPPORT GROUPS,
SUPPORT SYSTEMS

Lee, G.R. and Shehan, C.L. (1989). Social relations and the self-esteem of older persons. *Research on Aging, 11*(4), 427-442.

SECTION VII
SENIOR CENTERS, ADULT DAY CARE

Glenner, J., & Glenner, G.G. (1988/89). The crucible — Family dilemmas in Alzheimer's Disease: Day care — an alternative. *Activities, Adaptation & Aging, 13*(1/2), 1-23.
Krout, J. (1988). Senior center linkages with community organizations. *Research on Aging, 10*(2), 258-274.
Krout, J. (1988). The frequency, duration, and stability of senior center attendance. *Journal of Gerontological Social Work, 13*(1-2), 3-19.
Monk, A. & Cox, C. (1989, Nov.-Dec.). Integrating frail elderly into senior centers. *Perspective on Aging*, 24-25.

SECTION VIII
INTERGENERATIONAL PROGRAMS

SECTION IX
VOLUNTEERISM

SECTION X
EDUCATION, LEARNING, MEMORY, MEDIA USE

Dittman, J., & Redlin, M. (1989). Cheers for years: An educational fair to celebrate the older adult. *Lifelong Learning: An omnibus of Practice and Research*, *12*(4), 10-12.

Nebes, R. (1989). Semantic memory in Alzheimer's disease. *Psychological Bulletin*, *106*(3), 377-394.

Powers, W., Bacley-Hughes, B. and Ranft, M. (1989). Senior citizens as educational resources. *Educational Gerontology*, *15*(5), 481-488.

Ray, R.O. (1989). Informal learning in family caregiving: A worm's eye view. *Adult Education Quarterly*, *39*(1), 31-40.

Wacks, J., and Quinton, V. (1989). Life after death in the elder hostel classroom. *Lifelong Learning: An Omnibus of Practice and Research*, *12*(5), 23-24,28.

Weiss, C. (1989). TR and reminiscing: The pursuit of elusive memory and the art of remembering. *Therapeutic Recreation Journal*, *23*(3), 7-18.

SECTION XI
SUB-POPULATIONS, ETHNIC GROUPS,
CROSS-CULTURAL STUDIES, INTERNATIONAL ISSUES

Belgrave, L. (1988). The effects of race differences in work history, work attitudes, economic resources, and health on women's retirement. *Research on Aging*, *10*(3), 383-398.

Benefiel, P. (1988). Life satisfaction, leisure satisfaction, and leisure participation among Anglo, Black, and Hispanic older adults. Microform publications, University of Oregon.

Dyman, A.J. & Edwards, M.E. (1989). Reminiscence poetry groups: Sheepherding—A Navajo cultural tie that binds. *Activities, Adaptation & Aging*, *13*(4), 1-8.

Krain, M. and Trevino-Richard, T. (1987). Degree of dependency and racial differences in use of senior centers. *Phylon*, *48*(4), 299-308.

McCallum, J. (1988). Japanese Teinen Taishoku: How cultural values affect retirement. *Aging and Society*, *8*(1), 23-41.

Retsinas, J. and Garritz, P. (1988). The newly disabled: Blind nursing home residents. *Journal of Applied Gerontology*, 7(3), 367-388.

Romsa, G. and Blenman, M. (1989). Vacation patterns of the elderly German. *Annals of Tourism Research*, *16*(2).

Stull, D. and Scarisbrick-Hauser, A. (1989). Never married elderly: A reassessment with implications for long-term care policy. *Research on Aging*, *11*(1), 124-139.

Weinstein, L.B. (1989). Transcultural relocation: Adaptation of older americans to Israel. *Activities, Adaptation & Aging*, *13*(4), 33-42.

Wood, J. (1989). Communicating with older adults in health care settings: Cultural and ethnic consideration. *Educational Gerontology*, *15*(4), 351-362.

SECTION XII
ROLE OF PROFESSIONALS, PROFESSIONAL ISSUES, STAFF TRAINING, MANAGEMENT TECHNIQUES

Allen, C., Foto, M., More-Sperling, T. & Wilson, D. (1989, December). A medical review approach to Medicare outpatient documentation. *American Journal of Occupational Therapy*, *43*(12), 793-800.

Shaw, J. & Whelan, R. (1989, November). QA outcome measures in long term care. *J. Nurs Qual Assur*, 4(1), 48-61.

SECTION XIII
GOVERNMENT PUBLICATIONS

Note: The number given in these citations comes from the monthly catalogues which are arranged in numerical order starting in January. In the catalogue a description of the piece is given and the superintendent of documents number is listed which is necessary to retrieve the item from shelves.

U.S. Congress, Senate Special Committee on Aging. (1989). Aging America: Trends and projections. Washington, D.C.: Government Printing Office. 90-4342.

U.S. Congress, Senate Special Committee On Aging. (1990). Intergenerational educational partnerships: A lifetime of talent to share. Washington, D.C.: Government Printing Office. 90-5642.

U.S. Department of Health and Human Services, Public Health Service. (1989). Older and wiser: The Baltimore Longitudinal Study of Aging. Bethesda, Maryland, National Institutes of Health. 90-3829.

U.S. Department of State, Bureau of Consular Affairs. (1990). Travel tips for older Americans. Washington, D.C., Government Printing Office. 90-5447.

U.S. Health Resources and Services Administration. Bureau of Health Professions. (1989). Geriatric Activities. Rockville, Md., Bureau of Health Professions. 89-14283.

U.S. National Center for Health Statistics (1989). Physical functioning of the aged: U.S., 1984. Hyattsville, Md.: National Center for Health Statistics. 89-11543.

U.S. Superintendent of Documents. (1989). Aging (a bibliography). Washington, D.C.: Government Printing Office. 90-2402.

SECTION XIV
EXERCISE, WELLNESS,
PHYSICAL FITNESS ACTIVITIES

Clark, B. (1989, March). Tests for fitness in older adults: AAHPERD fitness task force. *Journal of Physical Education, Recreation and Dance*, *60*(3), 66-71.

Craig, B.W., Everhart, J. and Brown, R. (1989, August). Effects of progressive resistance training on growth hormone and testosterone levels in young and elderly subjects. *Mechanisms of Aging and Development*, *49*(2), 159-169.

Craig, B.W., Everhart, J. and Brown, R. (1989, August). The influence of high-resistance training on glucose tolerance in young and elderly subjects. *Mechanisms of Aging and Development*, *49*(2), 147-157.

Ekberg, J. (1990, February). Senior fitness: Getting into the swim of things. *Park and Recreation*, pp. 46-49.

Freysinger, V. (1990, January). A lifespan perspective on women and physical recreation. *Journal of Physical Education, Recreation and Dance*, *61*(1), 48-51.

Gard, S. (1989, December). Senior fitness: A runaway success. *Park and Recreation*, pp. 27-29.

Herbert, L., & Teague, M.L. (1988/89). Exercise adherence and older adults: A theoretical perspective. *Activities, Adaptation & Aging*, *13*(1/2), 91-105.

Matteson, M. (1989). Effects of a cognitive behavioral approach and positive reinforcement on exercise for older adults. *Educational Gerontology*, *15*(5), 497-514.

Mussleman, P.R. (1990, February). Hydrotherapy: Get the healing feeling. *Park and Recreation*, pp. 54-57,83.

Schnurr, P.P., Vaillant, C.O., and Vaillant, G.E. (1990). Predicting exercise in late midlife from young adult personality characteristics. *International Journal of Aging and Human Development*, *30*(2), 153-160.

Tappe, M. and Duda, J. (1988). Personal investment predictors of life satisfaction among physically active middle-aged and older adults. *The Journal of Psychology*, *122*(6), 557-566.

Teague, M.L. (1988/89). The 1990 PHS exercise objectives for older adults: Should they be changed. *Activities, Adaptation & Aging*, *13*(1/2), 107-116.

Weiss, J.C. (1988). The feeling great wellness program for older adults. *Activities, Adaptation & Aging*, *12*(3/4), 1-211.

SECTION XV
OTHER AND RELATED STUDIES

Abernathy, R.M. and Abdel-Ghany, M. (1989). Quality of goods and services as perceived by the elderly and the young/middle-adulthood consumers. *Lifestyles*, *10*(2), 123-138.

Bridge, N.J. and Gold, D. (1989). An analysis of the relationship between leisure and economics. *Journal of Leisurability*, *16*(2), 10-14.

Caldwell, L. and Adolph, S. (1989). Economic issues associated with disability: And then there is leisure. *Journal of Leisurability*, Vol. 16.

Cohen-Shalev, A. (1989). Old age style: Developmental changes in creative production from a life-span perspective. *Journal of Aging Studies*, *3*(1), 21-37.

Crawford, C. (1989). A view from sidelines: Disability, poverty and recreation in Canada. *Journal of Leisurability*, *16*(2), 3-9.

Dolinsky, A. and Rosenwaike, I. (1988). The role of demographic factors in the institutionalization of the elderly. *Research on Aging*, *10*(2), 235-257.

Ellis, R. and Oscar-Berman, M. (1989). Alcoholism, aging, and functional cerebral asymmetries. *Psychological Bulletin*, *106*(1), 128-147.

Ferrel, M. (1989). No income: No leisure. *Journal of Leisurability*, *16*(2), 15-16.

Hira, T.K., Fanslow, A.M., and Titus, P.M. (1989). Changes in financial status influencing level of satisfaction in households. *Lifestyles*, *10*(2), 107-122.

Kannisto, V. (1988). On the survival of centenarians and the span of life. *Population Studies*, *42*(3), 389-406.

Landry, J. (1989). Making leisure available in Dartmouth. *Journal of Leisurability*, *16*(1), 16-18.

Maypole, D.E. (1989). Alcoholism and the elderly: Review of theories, treatment and prevention. *Activities, Adaptation & Aging*, *13*(4), 43-54.

McCoin, J. (1988). Adult foster care, case management and quality of life: Interpretive literature review. *Adult Foster Care Journal*, *2*(2), 135-148.

Morgan, L. (1989). Planning for inclusion and support by reviewing a delivery system. *Journal of Leisurability*, *16*(1), 8-12.

Salisbury, T. (1989). Integration challenges: Surrey, British Columbia. *Journal of Leisurability*, *16*(1), 13-15.

Searle, M. (1988). The effects of selected economic factors on the leisure behavior of disabled and non-disabled older adults. *Journal of Leisurability*, *15*(1), 20-27.

Seltzer, M. (1989). Random and not so random thoughts on becoming and being a statistic: Professional and personal musings. *International Journal of Aging in Human Development*, *28*(1), 1-7.

Staff. (1988). Logos: Insidious messages or positive symbolism? *Journal of Leisurability*, *13*(3), 12-13.

Staff. (1988, August). Rhetoric or reform? No news is bad news. First report of the standing committee of the status of disabled persons. House of Commons. *Journal of Leisurability*, *16*(3), 3-8.

Staff. (1988). Twenty years since we put man on the moon: An interview with John Southern. *Journal of Leisurability*, *16*(3), 9-11.

Staff. (1988). Word choices – A lexicon of preferred terms for disability issues. (Ontario Office for Disabled Persons in conjunction with Advocacy groups). *Journal of Leisurability*, *16*(3), 14.

Stevenson, S. (1989). A test of peak load pricing on senior citizen recreationists: A case study of Steamboat Lake State Park. *Journal of Park and Recreation Administration*, *7*(1), 58-68.

Story, M. (1989). Knowledge and attitudes about the sexuality of older adults among retirement home residents. *Educational Gerontology*, *15*(5), 515-526.

Tedrick, T. (1989, Summer). Images of aging through leisure: From pluralistic ignorance to master status trait? *Journal of Leisurability*, *16*(3), 15-19.

Viney, L., Benjamin, Y. and Preston, C. (1988). Promoting independence in the elderly: The role of psychological, social, and physical constraints. *Clinical Gerontologist*, *8*(2), 3-17.

West, A. (1989). Recreation? If only I could afford it! *Journal of Leisurability*, *16*(2), 17-18.

9 781560 241324